CHILD AND ADOLESCENT PSYCHIATRY FOR THE SPECIALTY BOARD REVIEW

Third Edition

CHILD AND ADOLESCENT PSYCHIATRY FOR THE SPECIALTY BOARD REVIEW

Third Edition

Robert L. Hendren and Hong Shen

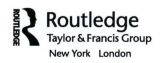

Routledge
Taylor & Francis Group
New York   London

Routledge
Taylor & Francis Group
270 Madison Avenue
New York, NY 10016

Routledge
Taylor & Francis Group
2 Park Square
Milton Park, Abingdon
Oxon OX14 4RN

© 2008 by Taylor & Francis Group, LLC
Routledge is an imprint of Taylor & Francis Group, an Informa business

Printed in the United States of America on acid-free paper
10 9 8 7 6 5 4 3 2

International Standard Book Number-13: 978-0-415-95598-0 (Softcover)

Visit the Taylor & Francis Web site at
http://www.taylorandfrancis.com

and the Routledge Web site at
http://www.routledge.com

DEDICATION

I appreciate the support and encouragement to update this book from my family, users of previous editions of this book, and Dr. Hong Shen. It has helped to keep me up to date.

RLH

Thanks to my dear wife, Ying Dong, for her love, understanding, and sacrifice during the revision of this book. A special thanks to my mentor, Dr. R. L. Hendren, for his encouragement, generous advice, and support.

HS

CONTENTS

Acknowledgment ix

Introduction. xi

References xiii

Part I: Multiple-Choice Questions

1 Normal Growth and Development 3

2 Developmental Disorders 21

3 Schizophrenia Spectrum Disorders and Affective Disorders 29

4 Disorders of Conduct and Behavior 39

5 Anxiety Disorders (Including Separation Anxiety, Overanxious and
Avoidant Disorders, Obsessive–Compulsive Disorder, Phobia, and
Posttraumatic Stress Disorder). 47

6 Eating and Nutritional Disorders. 55

7 Movement Disorders 63

8 Disorders of Somatic Function (Sleep, Elimination, Psychosomatic,
and Somatoform Disorders) 69

9 Substance Use and Abuse 77

10 Special Issues (Suicide, Sexuality, AIDS, Adjustment Disorder, Abuse,
Personality Disorders, Elective Mutism, and Stuttering) 85

11 Psychological Testing and Rating Scales. 97

12 Psychopharmacology. 103

13 Psychotherapies 115

14 Treatment Settings, Health-Care System, and Outcome. 123

15 Special Topics (Consultation, Forensics, and Public Health) 129

16 Research Design, Statistics, and Technologies 137

Part II: Mock Examination

17 Clinical Assessment, Differential Diagnosis, Formulation,
and Treatment Planning 147

18 Case Histories 155

ACKNOWLEDGMENT

A special acknowledgment goes to Stephanie Syphers for her contribution to the preparation of the manuscript and excellent secretarial and editorial assistance.

INTRODUCTION

Obtaining board certification in child and adolescent psychiatry represents a notable educational achievement as well as an important career credential. It also reflects the ability to prepare for and take comprehensive multiple-choice and oral examinations.

The purpose of this review book is to help guide candidates for subspecialty board certification in child and adolescent psychiatry from the American Board of Psychiatry and Neurology or certification in adolescent psychiatry from the American Society of Adolescent Psychiatry. It will also serve as a useful review for residents in training or for psychiatrists who desire to evaluate the currency of their knowledge in the field of child and adolescent psychiatry, especially when preparing for the recertification examination.

The book is divided into two parts, as are the board examinations. Part I consists of multiple-choice questions modeled after the types of questions on the actual examination. Part II is a mock examination based on the oral examination, but in multiple-choice format. These questions serve as an organizational guide for the oral examination and provide examples of the knowledge expected by the examiners.

Overall, the questions in this review book may be easier than the actual examination because the book is designed to serve a learning purpose. As with the actual examination, some of the answers may be controversial. In the actual examination, examiners also take the multiple-choice examination, and questions resulting in substantial disagreement are discarded. Child and adolescent psychiatry fellows and faculty have graciously reviewed this book, and the questions have been modified based on their comments.

In preparing for the board examinations, you may wish first to review this book and then to use the results to guide your studies, or you may complete a general review of child and adolescent psychiatry and then answer the board review questions, using the results to determine where you need additional study. You should review at least one comprehensive text in your preparation. Also, you should study the major journals publishing relevant material from the past 2 or 3 years, including the *Journal of the American Academy of Child and Adolescent Psychiatry,* the *American Journal of Psychiatry,* and the *Archives of General Psychiatry.* This should be done not only to obtain up-to-date information, but also to determine current areas of interest in the field as reflected in these major journals.

A good examination should do more than test knowledge; it should also be a learning experience and should help guide future knowledge acquisition. In this light, we hope that this review book not only will help you to organize your knowledge so that you pass the board examination, but also serve as a learning experience that benefits you and your patients.

REFERENCES

Note: With dramatic advances continually being made in the clinical sciences, it is a challenge for physicians to keep abreast of the modifications in treatment that such advances require and the new drugs being introduced each year. The authors and publisher of this volume have taken care to make certain that the doses of drugs and schedules of treatment are correct and compatible with standards generally accepted at the time of publication. However, it is essential for the reader to become fully cognizant of the information on the instruction inserts provided with each drug or therapeutic agent prior to administration or prescription.

Further, as some of the topics are by nature ambiguous, it is suggested that the reader consult the indicated reference sources for clarification should there be a discrepancy between the answer selected and that which appears in the book.

Each question, answer, and explanation can be found in one or more of the basic books on child and adolescent psychiatry, reference books, and published journal articles listed here. The references are cited by number, indicating the appropriate page numbers, with each appropriate answer in the text.

1. J. M. Wiener and M. K. Dulcan (Eds.). *Textbook of Child and Adolescent Psychiatry* (Third Edition). American Psychiatric Publishing, Inc., Arlington, VA, 2004.
2. M. K. Dulcan, D. R. Martini, and M. Lake. *Concise Guide to Child & Adolescent Psychiatry* (Third Edition). American Psychiatric Press, Washington, DC, 2003.
3. M. Lewis (Ed.). *Child and Adolescent Psychiatry: A Comprehensive Textbook* (Third Edition). Lippincott Williams & Wilkins, Philadelphia, PA, 2002.
4. *Diagnostic and Statistical Manual of Mental Disorders* (Fourth Edition Text Revision) (DSM-IV-TR). American Psychiatric Association, Washington, DC, 2000.

PART I

MULTIPLE-CHOICE QUESTIONS

1

NORMAL GROWTH AND DEVELOPMENT

QUESTIONS

Directions: Select the best response for each of the questions 1–67.

1. The development of the nervous system involves at least five major processes that are regulated in part by genetic factors and include all of the following *except:*

a. Differentiation of specific cell types
b. Immigration
c. Growth
d. Neural connectivity
e. Cell death

2. In contrast to the other developmental theories, reactive theories postulate that the child's development begins untouched by previous experience. The child then reacts to the environment. Examples of this type of theory include all of the following *except:*

a. Stimulus–response theory
b. Psychoanalysis
c. Learning theory
d. Operant conditioning
e. Classical conditioning

3. By the age of 3 years, most children can perform all of the following tasks *except:*

a. Run with ease
b. Copy a square
c. Copy a circle
d. Use a vocabulary of about 200 words
e. Use negative sentences and questions

4. Piaget postulated four stages of development. Which one of the following sequences of development describes the stages given by Piaget? (">" symbol = progression)

a. Concrete operational > sensorimotor > preoperational > formal operational
b. Preoperational > sensorimotor > concrete operational > formal operational
c. Sensorimotor > preoperational > formal operational > concrete operational
d. Sensorimotor > preoperational > concrete operational > formal operational
e. Sensorimotor > concrete operational > preoperational > formal operational

5. Building on Piaget's theories, Kohlberg suggested three major levels of moral development: (I) premorality, (II) morality of conventional role conformity, and (III) morality of self-accepted moral principles. He proposed two types in each level, going from type 1 as the lowest to type 6 as the highest. Which of the following statements best describes level II, type 3?

a. Punishment and obedience orientation
b. Agreement to obey only in return for some reward
c. Morality of social contract (democratically accepted law)
d. Conformity to the rules to please and gain approval (good-boy morality)
e. Commitment to universal ethical principles

6. Attachment is an affectional tie that one person forms to another person, binding them together in space and enduring over time. Examples of attachment behavior include all of the following *except:*

a. Promotion of proximity or contact
b. Crying and smiling
c. Looking and following
d. Vocalizing
e. Habituation

7. Most brain structures in the higher vertebrates have a larger number of neurons and synaptic connections during development than in adulthood. The name of the process by which the overproduction of synapses is decreased is called:

a. Extermination
b. Competitive elimination
c. Cell death
d. Enucleation
e. Trimming

8. Which one of the following neurotransmitter systems is thought to play an important role in sleep, mood, appetite, perception, and hormone secretion?

a. Serotonin (5-hydroxytryptamine, or 5-HT)
b. Dopamine (DA)
c. Norepinephrine (NE)
d. Acetylcholine (Ach)
e. Epinephrine

9. Which one of the following neurotransmitter systems has been shown to be critical in reward, in modulating movement, and in cognition?

a. Serotonin
b. Dopamine
c. Norepinephrine
d. Acetylcholine
e. Epinephrine

10. Which one of the following neurotransmitter systems modulates stress responses, central and peripheral arousal, and learning and memory?

a. Serotonin
b. Dopamine
c. Norepinephrine

d. Acetylcholine
e. Epinephrine

11. The precursor of serotonin is:

a. Phenylalanine
b. Tyrosine
c. Tryptophan
d. Choline
e. Histidine

12. Classic conditioning is *best* described by which one of the following phrases?

a. Behaviors that are strengthened or weakened as a function of the events that follow them.
b. Presentation or removal of an event after a response that increases the frequency of the response.
c. Removal of the reinforcing event after a response decreases the frequency of the previously reinforced response.
d. Certain stimuli coming to elicit reflex responses.
e. Reinforcing the response in the presence of one discrimination stimulus but not in the presence of another.

13. All of the following statements regarding behavior therapy/modification are correct *except:*

a. The techniques used are rooted in learning theory and the focus is on learned or acquired behavior.
b. Behavior can be altered through changes in the environmental influences.
c. Techniques should be administered only by highly trained professionals in clinical settings.
d. The approach can be used for different kinds of people with a variety of maladaptive behaviors and/or mental health problems.
e. There are three forms of learning including: classical conditioning, operant conditioning, and observational learning.

14. Which of the following statements regarding contemporary attachment theory is *not* an accurate description of the current theory?

a. Infants are predisposed from birth to respond socially to social partners as part of a survival-enhancing motivational system.
b. Infants develop security in their caregivers based on their prior experiences of sensitive, helpful, responsive care.
c. The security of attachment is shaped by reciprocal influences of each parent, the infant, and the environment.
d. Success in meeting early developmental challenges provides a strong or weak foundation for subsequent development.
e. There is a clear adaptive behavioral pattern in the infant and the parent that leads to a "secure" attachment.

15. Mary Ainsworth developed a research instrument known as the "strange situation" procedure to assess the security of attachment in infancy. In most middle-class samples, what proportion of infants is determined to be securely attached?

a. 10%
b. 40%
c. 65%
d. 80%
e. 90%

16. All of the following are memory strategies *except:*

a. Encoding and storage strategies
b. Rehearsal strategies
c. Perceptual strategies
d. Organizational strategies
e. Elaboration strategies

17. Which of the following structures mediate selective attachment?

a. Frontal lobes
b. Thalamus
c. Nucleus basalis of Meynert
d. Amygdala
e. Hippocampus

18. From approximately which of the following ages are children typically involved with sex play, such as "doctor" and "make a baby"?

a. 2 Years
b. 4 Years
c. 6 Years
d. 8 Years
e. 10 Years

19. At which of the following ages does a child identify himself or herself as a boy or a girl?

a. 12 to 18 Months
b. 2 to 3 Years
c. 4 to 5 Years
d. 6 to 7 Years
e. 7 to 8 Years

20. All of the following statements about the development of the cerebral cortex are accurate *except:*

a. Cortical neurons are acquired during the middle third of gestation.
b. A massive migration of neurons occurs during midgestation.
c. There are a larger number of neurons and axonal connections during adulthood than during early development.
d. Extrinsic (irradiation or viral infection) and intrinsic (genetic) factors can influence synapse stability and cause malformation.
e. Manipulation of sensory input can alter the structure and function of areas of the cortex.

21. All of the following are normal psychological reactions to acute illness in children *except:*

a. Increased attachment behavior
b. Regression
c. Excessive anxiety

d. Decreased competence

e. Passivity

22. Which of the following is a definition of assimilation as used by Piaget?

   a. A pattern of behavior in response to a range of external stimuli

   b. The broadening of a response to include a new, similar but not identical stimulus

   c. A modified response to a similar stimulus

   d. Changed responses centered on the infant's body

   e. Movement from an egocentric point of view

23. At what age is gender identity established?

   a. The first year of life

   b. Years 1 to 2

   c. Years 3 to 5

   d. Years 5 to 7

   e. Years 11 to 13

24. At what age range is gender role established?

   a. The first year of life

   b. Years 1 to 2

   c. Years 3 to 5

   d. Years 6 to 8

   e. Years 9 to 13

25. J. Tanner divided physical changes of puberty into stages. Which of the following sequences is correctly described for girls? (">" symbol = progression)

   a. Menarche (menstruation) > pubic hair > breast development

   b. Pubic hair > breast development > menarche

   c. Breast development > menarche > pubic hair

   d. Breast development > pubic hair > menarche

   e. Menarche > breast development > pubic hair

26. Which of the following developmental sequences correctly describes the Tanner staging for boys? (">" symbol = progression)

   a. Pubic hair > penile enlargement > ejaculation

   b. Axillary hair > testicular enlargement > penile enlargement

   c. Voice changes > pubic hair > ejaculation

   d. Penile enlargement > testicular enlargement > ejaculation

   e. Pubic hair > voice changes > penile enlargement

27. In general, studies of the effects of the timing of maturation in the United States suggest that early maturation is more advantageous for:

   a. Boys

   b. Girls

   c. Both boys and girls

   d. Neither boys nor girls

   e. Unknown since no clear pattern has changed

28. All of the following statements regarding neurotransmitter receptors are true except:

   a. Neurotransmitters and their metabolites have been measured in brain tissue, cerebrospinal fluid, plasma and blood elements, and urine.

   b. Modulator proteins often are associated with receptors.

   c. Benzodiazepines increase GABAergic (γ-aminobutyric acid-ergic) transmission in the brain, but do not bind directly to GABA receptors.

   d. Presynaptic receptors (autoreceptors) usually facilitate the release of the type of neurotransmitter that binds to them.

   e. Muscarinic receptors are found in the central nervous system.

29. All of the following are thought to be associated with serotonin transmission except:

   a. Slow-wave sleep

   b. Depression

   c. Thermoregulation

   d. Appetite regulation

   e. Prolactin secretion

30. Which of the following neurodevelopmental disorders is characterized by an extra X chromosome (i.e., XXY karyotype)?

   a. Fragile X syndrome

   b. Turner syndrome

   c. Klinefelter's syndrome

   d. Prader–Willi syndrome

   e. Wilson's disease

31. Margaret Mahler conceptualized an object relations framework to explain normal and deviant development. She described which of the following sequences of infant development? (">" symbol = progression)

   a. Symbiotic phase > autistic phase > separation –individuation

   b. Separation–individuation > autistic phase > symbiotic phase

   c. Symbiotic phase > separation–individuation > autistic phase

   d. Autistic phase > separation–individuation > symbiotic phase

   e. Autistic phase > symbiotic phase > separation–individuation

32. The following statements regarding the effects of culture and ethnicity on development are correct except:

   a. Culture can facilitate shaping and development of personality throughout life.

   b. The style of children's play can reflect the influence of cultural values.

   c. Child-rearing practices and peer influence can have effects on personality development.

   d. Facing contrasting cultural values, girls may experience greater difficulty and distress in shifting their values to the mainstream ones.

e. There are no differences in recognizing facial expressions among different cultural groups.

33. The following statements regarding the development of communication are correct *except:*

    a. A peak in the development of pragmatic skills occurs between the ages of 3 and 5 years.
    b. Young children use more decontextualized language in their storytelling.
    c. By age 2, children can tell stories, but rarely adhere to the original story line.
    d. By age 6, children have better narrative ability and adhere more to the story line.
    e. School-age children's storytelling is more sophisticated, providing information regarding causes of events.

34. Genetic studies that include young people have found the following *except:*

    a. There is evidence to support that genetics contribute to the etiology of attention-deficit hyperactivity disorder (ADHD).
    b. Several candidate genes have been studied and their association with ADHD is still controversial.
    c. Recent studies of Tourette's syndrome, chronic tics, and obsessive–compulsive disorder (OCD) suggest genetic transmission through an autosomal dominant mode.
    d. Autism is an autosomal dominant genetic disorder.
    e. Genetic factors play an important role in the etiology of dyslexia, although its exact mode of inheritance is still unknown.

35. Which one of the following concepts was used by Piaget to describe the preoperational child?

    a. Mastering the concept of conservation
    b. Abstract thinking
    c. Egocentrism
    d. Circular reactions
    e. Seriation and classification

36. Clinically, attachment theory is useful in all of the following circumstances *except:*

    a. Predicting the inevitable consequences/outcomes of early insecure attachment
    b. Understanding the nature of development of child psychopathology
    c. Understanding child abuse/neglect
    d. Understanding delinquency
    e. Treatment of mental illnesses in childhood

37. The transactional model of development, based on recent research data in infancy, has largely supplanted drive theory's fixation-regression model (main effects model). Which of the following descriptions applies to the main effects model?

    a. Dynamic ongoing transactions between the individual and the environment
    b. Plasticity of human development

c. Continuing and mutually reciprocal interactions between the child and the parent
d. Critical periods concept
e. An individual characteristic is predisposed by genetic factors and heritablity

38. Temperament is viewed as individual differences in the behavioral style that individuals utilize in different situations. Which of the following statements about temperament is not accurate?

    a. Measures of temperament include activity level, rhythmicity, and approach–withdrawal.
    b. Temperament can be categorized into three constellations: easy, difficult, and slow to warm up.
    c. The stability of these traits increases with increasing age.
    d. Early characterization of temperament in infancy is invariably predictive of temperament at each successive stage.
    e. Genetic factors contribute to temperament.

39. The dysfunction of the hypothalamic–pituitary–adrenal (HPA) axis neuroendocrine pathway may be related to the following childhood psychiatric and behavioral disorders/conditions *except:*

    a. Major depressive disorder (MDD)
    b. Posttraumatic stress disorder (PTSD)
    c. Childhood autism
    d. Psychosocial dwarfism
    e. Childhood shyness

40. Strategies employed in biological psychiatry include all of the following techniques *except:*

    a. Measurement of neurotransmitters, metabolites, and neurotransmitter-related enzymes and measurement of neurotransmitter receptors
    b. Studying genetic factors and environmental factors
    c. Studying the mechanisms of psychological defenses
    d. Neuroendocrine studies
    e. Brain-imaging studies

41. Maturational brain changes include all of the following *except:*

    a. Progressive increases in brain weight
    b. Increased cerebral cortical thickness
    c. Progression of regional myelination
    d. Increase in the neuronal density in the cerebral cortex
    e. Critical importance of prefrontal cortex development

42. Initiation of neurotransmission is accomplished by all of the following actions *except:*

    a. Release of presynaptic neurotransmitter
    b. Binding of the neurotransmitter to the presynaptic receptor
    c. Binding of the neurotransmitter to the postsynaptic receptor
    d. Activation of postsynaptic receptor
    e. Regulation of the second messenger system

43. All of the following statements regarding the function of the basal ganglia are correct *except:*
    a. They modulate motor and some autonomic functions.
    b. They are involved in intellectual functions.
    c. They may be involved in the etiology of obsessive–compulsive disorder (OCD).
    d. They may be involved in the etiology of ADHD.
    e. They can initiate particular movements.

44. All of the following statements regarding temperament are correct *except:*
    a. Children with easy temperaments possess biological regularity, adapting quickly and positively to changes.
    b. Children with difficult temperaments possess biological irregularity, adapting to changes in a stressful and distressing manner.
    c. Children with slow-to-warm-up temperaments possess withdrawal tendencies, adapting to changes slowly.
    d. All children can fit into one of the three groups listed in a, b, or c.
    e. Integration between environment and temperament is important in a healthy or pathologic psychological development.

45. Nearly all of the brain-behavior syndromes in children—such as attention deficit hyperactivity disorder, learning and language disorders, autism, and schizophrenia—show a markedly higher incidence in boys. Possible biological correlations include all of the following *except:*
    a. Smaller frontal lobe proportionally to other parts of the brain in boys than in girls
    b. Less complete development of dominance in girls
    c. Lesser hemispheric size differences in girls
    d. Androgen sensitivity in boys
    e. Greater vulnerability to brain damage in boys

46. All of the following statements regarding securely attached infants are true *except:*
    a. Influences on attachment include the reciprocal influences of each parent.
    b. A secure attachment, once formed, remains stable over the first 2 years.
    c. The goodness of fit of the temperaments of both parents and the infant influences attachment.
    d. Changes in attachment, if they occur at all, can occur at predictable times.
    e. Research evidence very weakly supports the association between secure attachment and personality organization.

47. Reasons for a young child's behaving insecurely in a strange situation (e.g., day care) include all of the following *except:*
    a. Confidence of having accessible caregivers
    b. An insecure attachment
    c. Cultural variations
    d. Insensitivity of maternal care
    e. Instability in the infant's environment

48. All of the following statements regarding fathers' relationships with their children have been validated in general population studies in the current literature *except:*
    a. Fathers engage in care-taking activities less than mothers.
    b. Mothers and fathers engage in different types of interactions with their children.
    c. Mothers are more sensitive to their children's characteristics and needs.
    d. Fathers have less confidence in their parenting abilities.
    e. Infants respond similarly to both maternal and paternal interactive styles.

49. All of the following statements regarding the development of attention are accurate *except:*
    a. Motivation has a strong effect on attention.
    b. Between ages 5 and 7, the child's attention is stimulus bound.
    c. Social class has a powerful effect on the attention of preschool children.
    d. Measures of sustained attention, reaction time, and motor inhibition show the largest increases between 4 and 6 years of age.
    e. Attachment may have an effect on attention.

50. Deviant speech or language production or a lack of comprehension may result in all of the following *except:*
    a. Learning difficulties/disorders
    b. Low intelligence
    c. Poor self-esteem and social isolation
    d. Academic impairment
    e. Behavioral problems

51. In which of the following ways is the genital self-stimulation of girls different from that of boys?
    a. It begins earlier.
    b. The format is more constant.
    c. Girls use more indirect techniques.
    d. Masturbation always results in pleasure.
    e. Girls show less overt disturbance or anxiety.

52. Which of the following correctly describes the father's role in child development?
    a. Fathers are more involved than mothers in rearing their children.
    b. Fathers are less likely to play with their children.
    c. Fathers' involvement helps the establishment of gender identity and role.
    d. Daughters of more actively involved fathers are more masculine.
    e. Sons of more actively involved fathers are more feminine.

53. Gender identity relates to all of the following *except:*
    a. A child's sense of being male or female
    b. The etiology of gender identity disorder (transsexualism)
    c. A child's capacity to categorize men and women by gender

d. The etiology of homosexual attraction

e. Stability throughout life span with some exceptions

54. All of the following statements accurately describe the development of adolescence *except:*

a. Girls start puberty approximately 2 years earlier than boys.

b. With dramatic growth in cognitive ability, adolescents can reach the stage of formal operations.

c. More girls perceive themselves as being overweight than boys.

d. Loss of cortical synapses during adolescence is called "pruning."

e. Authoritative parenting style is associated with adolescents' incompetence and negative outcomes.

55. All of the following could result in amenorrhea in girls *except:*

a. Extensive exercise

b. Endocrine disorders

c. Restricted diets

d. Stress

e. Hypothalamic hypergonadism

56. All of the following statements regarding adolescent homosexuality are accurate based on the current state of our knowledge *except:*

a. Homosexual contacts are most frequent in early adolescence.

b. Homosexual contact in adolescence does not necessarily lead to a homosexual identification.

c. There is a strong genetic component to homosexuality.

d. Homosexual men are more likely to be born as the oldest son.

e. Homosexuality may be associated with neurosteroids.

57. All of the following statements regarding adolescence are correct *except:*

a. The majority of teenagers (approximately 80%) do not experience marked turmoil or psychological disturbance.

b. Only a minority of adolescents develop major mood disorders.

c. A Centers for Disease Control (CDC) survey of high school students in 2000 indicated a very low rate of suicidal ideation.

d. Girls are more likely than boys to experience emotional disturbance.

e. Adolescents have greater mood variability than adults.

58. All of the following statements regarding adolescence are correct *except:*

a. Reaching Tanner stage III was associated with increasing depression in boys.

b. There are age-related changes in the balance of dopamine regulation, which lead to changes in the adolescent's reward system.

c. Adolescents' risk-taking behavior is associated with a high rate of accidental death.

d. Variation of risk-taking behavior exists among different age groups.

e. Arnett proposed a concept—"emerging adulthood"—to capture the late teens through the early 20s.

59. All of the following statements regarding parents of adolescents are correct *except:*

a. Parents of adolescents should use qualitatively different boundaries than those with younger children.

b. Fathers of bulimic teenagers were rated as less affectionate and more controlling.

c. Parents may experience psychological changes as their adolescent children develop.

d. Parents of reconstituted families face different developmental tasks compared to those of nuclear families.

e. Adoptive families with adolescents may follow a psychological pathway similar to that of other nuclear families.

60. At what age do children first start to understand the irreversibility of death?

a. Younger than 1 year of age

b. 1 to 2 Years of age

c. 3 to 5 Years of age

d. School-age children

e. Middle adolescence

61. All of the following statements regarding development and a cognitive–behavioral therapy (CBT) approach are correct *except:*

a. CBT is an integration of behavioral models with a cognitively mediated model.

b. According to Beck, cognition may consist of cognitive structure (cognitive schema), cognitive content, cognitive processes, and cognitive products.

c. According to Beck, people have their own schemas through which they view themselves, others, and the world in unique ways.

d. Dysfunctional schema and biased interpretation can result in psychopathology.

e. Youth with ADHD tend to misperceive threats and demands of the environment, making attributional errors.

62. Cross-cultural studies that support the important role of culture in shaping personality have demonstrated all of the following findings *except:*

a. Japanese infants are raised more interdependently than are American infants.

b. White children demonstrate a stronger sense of external control than do Black children in the United States.

c. American parents emphasize independence to a greater extent than do parents in other cultures.

d. Competitive striving is highly valued among Native American children as compared with "Anglo" children.

e. Asian mothers have more confidence in their children's academic ability than do mothers in the United States.

63. Which one of the following enzymes is the rate-limiting enzyme responsible for the synthesis of serotonin?

    a. Tyrosine hydroxylase
    b. Tryptophan hydroxylase
    c. Monoamine oxidase (MAO)
    d. Catecholamine-O-methyltransferase (COMT)
    e. Dopamine hydroxylase

64. Which of the following is the metabolite of serotonin?

    a. Vanillylmandelic acid (VMA)
    b. Homovanillic acid (HVA)
    c. 3-Methoxy-4-hydroxyphenylglycol (MHPG)
    d. 5-Hydroxyindoleacetic acid (HIAA)
    e. 3,4-Dihydrophenylacetic acid (DOPAC)

65. Which of the following neurotransmitter systems has been shown to modulate attention, novelty seeking, and memory through basal forebrains to the limbic system and cortex?

    a. Serotonergic neurotransmission
    b. GABAergic neurotransmission
    c. Dopaminergic neurotransmission
    d. Cholinergic neurotransmission
    e. Glutamatergic neurotransmission

66. Which of the following neurotransmission systems is crucial for inhibiting excitatory neurons?

    a. Serotonergic neurotransmission
    b. GABAergic neurotransmission
    c. Dopaminergic neurotransmission
    d. Cholinergic neurotransmission
    e. Glutamatergic neurotransmission

67. Which of the following neurotransmission systems is crucial for forming of memory?

    a. Serotonergic neurotransmission
    b. GABAergic neurotransmission
    c. Dopaminergic neurotransmission
    d. Cholinergic neurotransmission
    e. Glutamatergic neurotransmission

Matching

68–71. Match each stage of development with one of the following development tasks:

    a. Greater physical independence
    b. Adaptation to the outside world
    c. Defining one's own self
    d. Greater separation and demands

68. Infancy

69. 1.5 to 3 years

70. School age

71. Adolescence

72–75. Match each term used by Freud to describe a developmental stage with one of the following corresponding descriptive terms used by Erikson:

    a. Identity
    b. Autonomy
    c. Basic trust
    d. Initiative

72. Oral

73. Anal

74. Phallic

75. Adolescence

76–79. For each of the brain regions listed, select from the following functions that which most closely describes the brain region's actions:

    a. Maintaining and regulating motor and information flow
    b. Motor and executive functions
    c. Incoming information modulation
    d. Emotional and memory functions

76. Frontal lobe

77. Temporal lobe

78. Basal ganglia

79. Reticular system

80–85. For each of the named major figures in developmental psychiatry, choose from the following terms or descriptions that which is most associated with his or her theory:

    a. Transitional object
    b. Attachment theory
    c. Assimilation, accommodation
    d. Developmental lines
    e. Reparation
    f. Goodness of fit

80. Bowlby

81. Piaget

82. Winnicott

83. Melanie Klein

84. Chess and Thomas

85. Anna Freud

86–101. Match each defense mechanism listed with one of the following examples that best describes it:

    a. An adolescent "forgets" to tell her parents about a failing grade in school.
    b. An adolescent who is angry with a teacher berates a sibling for no apparent reason.
    c. An adolescent denies any feeling of abandonment or rejection by the noncustodial parent after a divorce.
    d. An adolescent returns to childish and dependent behavior following a family move to a new city.
    e. An adolescent mother resents the demands that caring for her child make on her. However, she repeatedly tells herself and others how wonderful motherhood is. At times, she worries unnecessarily that some harm will come to her child.

f. An adolescent experiencing repeated trouble with the law claims that all of the problems are the fault of law enforcement officers, who have it in for him.

g. An adolescent with a terminal illness volunteers to work as a hospital aide.

h. When asked about the automobile accident in which his father was killed, an adolescent begins discussing the mechanics of trauma, velocity of impact, safety rules, and changing trends in life expectancy.

i. An adolescent, in a cool, unemotional manner, describes the circumstances of a serious automobile accident in which he received multiple injuries.

j. A hospitalized adolescent views each member of the medical staff as being all "good" or all "bad."

k. An adolescent repeatedly engages in risk-taking behavior.

l. An adolescent laughs about an embarrassing encounter with a teacher.

m. An adolescent explains her drug abuse by saying that "everybody" does it.

n. An adolescent girl who is angry at her family after being grounded runs away from home without verbally expressing her anger.

o. An adolescent identifies with a rock star or an athletic coach whom he admires.

p. An adolescent whose father recently died of a myocardial infarction begins a vigorous exercise program.

86. Denial

87. Projection

88. Splitting

89. Acting out

90. Regression

91. Counterphobia

92. Identification

93. Reaction formation

94. Repression

95. Displacement

96. Isolation of affect

97. Rationalization

98. Intellectualization

99. Sublimation

100. Humor

101. Altruism

102–104. For each of the brain regions listed, select from the following the neurotransmitter that is most associated with it:

a. Dopamine
b. Serotonin
c. Norepinephrine

102. Locus ceruleus

103. Substantia nigra

104. Raphe nuclei

ANSWERS AND EXPLANATIONS

1. (b) All of the major processes listed are involved in the morphogenesis of the nervous system except "immigration," which is not a term used in cell growth. "Migration" is the term used and is the fifth major process referred to in the question. *(Ref. 3, p. 6)*

2. (b) The structural theory of psychoanalysis as well as the theories of Erikson and Piaget suggest that there is a genetically determined capacity for the development of patterns, or systems of behaviors, so that the child acts on the environment from the beginning. The clinical implication is that some kind of reorganization within the child is necessary for change to occur. The clinical implication of the reactive theories is that since symptoms are learned behavior, the symptom is removed through relearning or environmental change. These theories include stimulus–response theory, learning theory, classical conditioning theory, and operant conditioning theory. *(Ref. 1, pp. 16–17)*

3. (b) By the age of 3 years, children can run with ease, although not with great skill. A child at 2 can copy a circle; by age 3, a cross; by age 5, a square; and by age 7, a diamond. Vocabulary gradually increases to about 200 words by age 2. Between ages 2 and 3 years, children start using negative sentences and questions. *(Ref. 1, pp. 17, 19; Ref. 3, pp. 246–247)*

4. (d) Four major stages are described by Piaget. They are (1) a sensorimotor stage (0 though 18–24 months); (2) a preoperational stage (2 through 7 years); (3) a stage of concrete operations (6–7 through 11 years); and a stage of formal operations (11 years to adulthood). *(Ref. 1, pp. 20–22; Ref. 3, pp. 174–176)*

5. (d) Kohlberg's levels are as follows *(Ref. 1, pp. 28–29; Ref. 3, pp. 265–266)*:

Level I. Premorality
  Type 1. Punishment and obedience orientation
  Type 2. Agreement to obey in return for reward
Level II. Morality of conventional role conformity
  Type 3. Good-boy morality
  Type 4. Authority-maintaining morality
Level III. Morality of self-accepted moral principles
  Type 5. Morality of democratically accepted law
  Type 6. Morality of individual principles of conscience

6. (e) Attachment behavior includes crying, smiling, vocalizing, looking, following, approaching, embracing, clinging, and grasping. Attachment behavior is terminated because either the desired response has been achieved or the response becomes habituated or extinguished. *(Ref. 1, pp. 29–30; Ref. 3, pp. 164–165)*

7. (b) Studies of a variety of mammalian species support the hypothesis that competitive interactions between two or more populations of neurons early in development play a significant role in the elimination of the initial population of axons and in the later segregation of their synapses. Competitive elimination is also referred to as pruning. *(Ref. 3, p. 38)*

8. (a) Serotonin (or 5-HT) is thought to play an important role in all of the processes listed. In addition, serotonin is thought to be an impulse modulator and is involved with sexual activity. See questions 9–11 to learn the role of the other neurotransmitters listed. *(Ref. 3, p. 47)*

9. (b) Dopamine has been shown to be critical in modulating movement and cognition, and in modulating behavioral activation, novelty seeking, and reward. *(Ref. 3, pp. 48–49)*

10. (c) Noradrenergic neurons critically modulate all of the functions listed. *(Ref. 3, pp. 48–49)*

11. (c) Tryptophan is the precursor of serotonin. Tyrosine is the precursor of dopamine and norepinephrine. *(Ref. 3, pp. 48–49)*

12. (d) Classical conditioning is concerned with stimuli (such as noise, light, taste) that evoke involuntary or automatic responses. Answer **(a)** is a definition of operant conditioning; operants have some influence (operate) on the environment. Answer **(b)** is a definition of reinforcement, answer **(c)** is a definition of extinction, and answer **(e)** is a definition of stimulus control; all are basic principles of operant conditioning. *(Ref. 3, pp. 155–157)*

13. (c) Behavioral therapy is based on the learning theory, focusing on behaviors that are learned. Both adaptive and maladaptive behaviors can be modified and reshaped through learning process and changes in environmental influences. This approach can be used in different settings and for different populations including children and adolescents. There are three forms of learning as listed in answer **e** that are considered as the roots of behavior therapy. *(Ref. 3, pp. 154–155)*

14. (e) Contrary to the view that evolutionary processes have equipped infants with a single adaptive attachment pattern (i.e., "secure attachment") that is based on a species-specific style of sensitive parental care, different patterns of infant attachment behavior can be considered adaptive in different care-giving contexts and in relation to differing parental styles. *(Ref. 3, pp. 164–165)*

15. (c) The majority (approximately 65%) of infants in middle-class families are securely attached. Securely attached infants are more autonomous, symbolic, and ego resilient than are infants whose attachment is rated as anxious resistant or anxious avoidant. *(Ref. 3, p. 166)*

16. (c) Preschool children learn or memorize using nonverbal strategies, such as pointing and looking (encoding and storage). Growing older, children can use more complex strategies, such as rehearsal and organizational strategies. To enhance storage, children can add meaning to the presented items (elaboration). Gradually they can more efficiently store and retrieve information by selectively using different strategies. Perceptual strategies are not memory strategies. *(Ref. 3, p. 232)*

17. **(e)** Sensory data are conveyed to the hippocampus, where the data are evaluated for novelty, salience, and emotional importance. The thalamus is involved in sensory processing, local sensorimotor integration, memory, emotion, attention, and alerting. The nucleus basalis of Meynert is involved with memory. The amygdala is involved with control, spontaneity, and flexibility of affect and cognition. *(Ref. 3, pp. 126–127, 234)*

18. **(b)** At age 2 years, children are interested in toilets and the sensation of defecation (anal eroticism). Between age 2 and 3 years, they become more interested in urination, even playing with the urinary stream. Around the same age, they may touch each other's genitals while taking a bath together. Around age 4, children may engage in sex play using themes and assigning roles, such as "doctor" and "make a baby." After age 4 or 5, their sexual activity becomes more secretive and sex play decreases in the early school years. *(Ref. 3, p. 280)*

19. **(b)** A child's basic sense of self as male or female is defined as gender identity that typically appears around age 2 or 3 years. Children begin to identify themselves or categorize others by sex based on hair or clothing. In the past, "the earlier the better" approach was used to determine the time for sex reassignment surgery for children with ambiguous genitals, but recent studies question this approach. *(Ref. 1, p. 813; Ref. 3, pp. 274–275)*

20. **(c)** Neurons as well as their axons and dendrites are more numerous only during a well-defined period of early development. Environmental and intrinsic factors influence the development of the cortex, which has a remarkable amount of plasticity. *(Ref. 3, pp. 22–42)*

21. **(d)** Many factors can influence a child's reactions to his or her illness, or that of a family member, including age, premorbid psychopathology, severity and course of the illness, etc. In addition to increased attachment behavior, regression, excessive anxiety, and passivity, a normal child may manifest biopsychological symptoms, frightening fantasies, and reactivation of premorbid conditions in response to acute illness. In contrast, decreased competence usually occurs when a child reacts to a chronic illness, not an acute one. *(Ref. 1, pp. 38–39)*

22. **(b)** Answer (**a**) is a definition of schema, answer **c** is a definition of accommodation, and answer (**d**) is a definition of primary circular reactions. Answer (**e**) is a definition of decentration and, while it is an example of accommodation, answer (**b**) is a more concise definition. *(Ref. 1, pp. 20–21; Ref. 3, pp. 174–175)*

23. **(b)** The biological determination of sex occurs before birth; however, gender identity is influenced by social and cultural factors, and is usually established by 1 or 2 years of age. By 2.5 years, children can categorize people by sex and recognize their own sex. Gender identity disorders become evident in the preschool years. *(Ref. 1, p. 813; Ref. 3, p. 275)*

24. **(c)** Gender role refers to a set of adopted behaviors that are either typically male or female. People can recognize a child to be primarily male or female based on those behaviors.

Gender role is usually established between ages 3 and 5, with girls being more malleable than boys. *(Ref. 1, p. 813; Ref. 3, p. 275)*

25. **(d)** In girls, puberty begins with breast bud development, followed by the growth of pubic hair, and finally by the onset of menstruation. The timing of each physical characteristic relative to the others can vary from individual to individual. For girls, puberty begins and ends about 1.5 years earlier than for boys. *(Ref. 1, pp. 32–34; Ref. 3, pp. 333–334)*

26. **(a)** In boys, puberty begins with the growth of pubic hair and penile and testicular enlargement, followed by axillary hair, and then voice changes, facial hair growth, and ejaculation. Puberty has been beginning earlier for both boys and girls during the past century, probably as the result of improvements in nutrition and health. *(Ref. 1, pp. 32–34; Ref. 3, pp. 333–334)*

27. **(a)** In the United States, early maturation is more advantageous socially for boys and middle or later maturation is advantageous socially for girls as girls are exposed to greater stress from peers and parents from early development, whereas boys experience a greater stress from their peers when they develop late. Cultural values attached to the meaning of early and late maturation do have an effect. *(Ref. 3, p. 334)*

28. **(d)** Presynaptic receptors usually inhibit the release of the neurotransmitter that binds to them. Benzodiazepines bind to separate receptors that are linked to certain GABA receptors. Modulator proteins are frequently interposed between neurotransmitter receptors and effectors, which may modify synaptic function. Both muscarinic and nicotinic receptors are present in the central nervous system of humans. *(Ref. 3, pp. 46–52, 944–949)*

29. **(e)** Serotonin is believed to be involved in thermoregulation, the genesis of rapid-eye-movement (REM) sleep, as well as slow-wave sleep. Prolactin secretion is inhibited by dopamine and is not related to serotonin. *(Ref. 3, p. 47–48)*

30. **(c)** Among listed neurodevelopment disorders, only male patients with Klinefelter syndrome carry a karyotype of XXY and have deficits in cognition and language and learning difficulties. *(Ref. 1, pp. 186–187)*

31. **(e)** Mahler described object relations from normal autistic phase to symbiotic phase, followed by the separation–individuation (including four subphases: differentiation, practicing, rapprochement, and object constancy). Her theory has been criticized recently as pathologizing normal infancy. *(Ref. 1, p. 34; Ref. 3, p. 461)*

32. **(e)** Culture consists of a set of values, behaviors, beliefs, and attitudes that are shared by a group of people, and shape their personality development from childhood through adulthood. Children may grow up in a more interdependent or independent culture and their play reflects their cultural values. Parenting styles and peer influence can certainly affect children's personality development. Adapting and shifting between cultural values (especially for immigrants moving from their original culture to a new one) are considered as acculturation. Conflicting cultural values may delay the process of acculturation. Girls experience more difficulties and distress in this process, which can lead to disruption of personality development.

Studies show differences in recognition of facial expressions (such as sadness and anger) among different cultural groups. *(Ref. 3, pp. 494–496)*

33. **(b)** Children live very much in the present and their storytelling reflects this. Between ages 3 and 5 there is rapid development of pragmatic skills with increasing language to describe events and incidents. Younger children's storytelling is not structured or organized, is mostly collections of random events, and rarely refers to events outside the immediate context. As age progresses, more sophisticated storytelling occurs, which is associated with acquisition of literacy and cognitive development. *(Ref. 3, pp. 248–250)*

34. **(d)** Studies support the genetic habitability of ADHD, dyslexia, Tourette's disorder, and OCD and genetic factors are thought to play important roles in their etiology. Many candidate genes have been identified and investigated, with mixed results, some of which showed strong associations. Although evidence supports an autosomal dominant inheritance for Tourette's, chronic tics, and OCD, the genetic mechanism of inheritance of autism is still inconclusive. *(Ref. 3, pp. 417–427)*

35. **(c)** The preoperational child is characterized by Piaget as having two substages: the substage of symbolic activity (2 to 4 years old) and the substage of decentration (4 to 7 years old). The preoperational child is extremely egocentric. The concept of circular reactions was used by Piaget in the sensorimotor stage. Children are not capable of mastering the concepts of conservation, classification, and seriation until the stage of concrete operational stage. The ability to think abstractly does not fully appear until the stage of formal operations. *(Ref. 1, pp. 20–22; Ref. 3, pp. 173–176)*

36. **(a)** Clinical studies of attachment are helpful in understanding most of the situations listed. Insecure attachment can potentially foreshadow later development problems; however, the outcomes may be influenced by many factors and may not be necessarily fixed or inevitable. *(Ref. 3, pp. 169–170)*

37. **(d)** The main effects model describes critical and sensitive periods emphasizing the great importance of early experience. Having never been empirically substantiated, the main effects model was replaced by Sameroff's transactional model, which emphasizes the importance of mutual effects between the child and the parents' characteristics. More recent research on the development of infancy supports the view that the course of development is codetermined by both biological adaptation and experience, and both genetic and environmental factors influence development, as described by the other answers given in this question. *(Ref. 3, pp. 293–295)*

38. **(d)** Measures of temperament developed by Chess and Thomas that are often used include activity level, rhythmicity, approach–withdrawal, adaptability, responsiveness, intensity of reactions, quality of mood, distractibility, and attention span. They proposed three constellations of temperament, including easy temperament, difficult temperament, and slow-to-warm-up temperament. Genetic factors that contribute to temperament include emotionality, activity, and sociability. While temperamental traits often continue unchanged into adulthood, there are occasions where temperament is modified by such factors as the family and environment. *(Ref. 1, p. 35; Ref. 3, pp. 220–224)*

39. **(d)** Neuroendocrine influence in early stages of development can be long-lasting and permanent. The HPA axis is one neuroendocrine pathway (among others, such as the somatotrophic axis, hypothalamic–pituitary–thyroid axis, and hypothalamic–pituitary–gonadal axis) that may play important roles in regulating brain development. All the listed conditions can be related to the dysfunction of the HPA axis except for the psychosocial dwarfism believed to be associated with the hyposecretion of growth hormone (a dysfunction of the somatotropic axis). *(Ref. 3, pp. 93–111)*

40. **(c)** All of the strategies listed are employed in biological psychiatry except for answer **(c)**. Both genetic and environmental factors are interrelated and influential, and should be considered within the realm of biological psychiatry. *(Ref. 3, pp. 46–47)*

41. **(d)** From infancy to adulthood, there are progressive increases in brain weight, head circumference, and cerebral cortical thickness, and a progressive decrease in neuronal density in the cerebral cortex and other cortical and subcortical regions. Most tracts are myelinated by the age of 3 years, but some are not until adulthood. Because of being associated with stages of cognitive development, prefrontal cortex changes are critically important. *(Ref. 3, pp. 60–61)*

42. **(b)** The initiation of transmission is accompanied by (1) the release of presynaptic neurotransmitter; (2) the binding of the neurotransmitter to postsynaptic receptors; (3) the activation of receptors; and/or (4) the regulation of secondary messengers. The termination of the transmission is the result of (1) ending of the excitation of the presynaptic terminal; (2) depletion of the neurotransmitter; (3) binding of the neurotransmitter to the presynaptic receptors, which turns off the release of the neurotransmitter; (4) reuptake of the neurotransmitter by the presynaptic terminal; and/or (5) metabolism by extracellular enzymes, which depletes the neurotransmitter available in the synaptic cleft. *(Ref. 3, pp. 48–49, 944, 949)*

43. **(e)** The basal ganglia, consisting of five subcortical interconnected parts (caudate nucleus, putamen, globus pallidus, subthalamic nucleus, and the ventral mesencephalic dopamine system), play an important role in maintaining and regulating motor and some autonomic functions through their connections/circuits to the cortex. It is also believed that the dysfunction of the basal ganglia and/or their associated circuits is involved in some neuropsychiatric conditions (especially conditions related to motor and attention dysfunctions) such as Parkinson's disease, OCD, and ADHD. The basal ganglia appear to be participating by enabling particular movements and controlling their sequencing, rather than directly initiating their occurrence. *(Ref. 3, p. 126)*

44. **(d)** In the New York Longitudinal Study, Chess and Thomas proposed three categories of temperament, with approximately 40% of the study population having an easy temperament, approximately 10% having a difficult temperament, and approximately 15% having a temperament that is slow to warm up. Some of the children did not fit into any one of those three

groups, but rather they manifested a combination of temperament traits, representing the variations of normal limits. The goodness or poorness of fit is a concept the researchers used to describe the level of integration between temperament and environment. *(Ref. 3, pp. 221–223)*

45. **(a)** Answer **a** is incorrect and irrelevant. The remaining answers describing differences between the developing brains of boys and of girls all reflect gender differences that place boys at a greater risk of emotional disturbance. Research on androgen sensitivity in the development of sexual preference and gender identity, and on the development of aggressiveness and activity level, also indicates differences between the sexes. Recent imaging and autopsy studies support that unilateral changes in certain brain regions (rather than the asymmetry of the brain) may be a possible explanation of some learning disorders. *(Ref. 3, pp. 126–128)*

46. **(b)** While the quality of early care is an important influence on attachment, other important influences include the care-giving involvement of the father, marital harmony, socioeconomic stress, the infant's own temperament, and the fit of this temperament with the temperaments of the parents. The security of attachment may remain relatively stable but it can change during the second year of life. When such changes occur, they are predictably linked to changes in the primary caregiver–infant relationship. While secure attachment has long-lasting implications for later development, research data only weakly support its association with personality development because the influence seems to wane over time, and other influences may also play a role in developing self-concept and personality organization. *(Ref. 3, pp.167–169)*

47. **(a)** Clearly, an increased fear response to a strange situation could be due to an insecure attachment and/or insecurity of maternal care. Research has also shown that an insecure reaction in a strange situation can be due to cultural and subcultural normal variations and to the emotional climate of the environment around the child. The strange situation procedure originally designed for middle-class infants in the United States cannot be used appropriately or validly to assess an infant's security of attachment across different ethnic groups. In a securely attached situation, children have confidence that their caregivers can be accessed for assistance and will meet their needs. *(Ref. 3, pp. 166–168)*

48. **(e)** Fathers today are more engaged and accessible than previously, but mothers still engage in daily care-taking and nurturing activities more than fathers. Mothers develop more "on the job" parenting skills, and thus are more sensitive to their children's needs. Psychologically, fathers are prepared differently than mothers before the birth of the child, and they may have low self-esteem and feel inadequate to be a provider. Mothers and fathers engage in different types of interaction with their children. Interestingly, infants also respond differently to their parents' interactive styles. *(Ref. 3, pp. 289–291)*

49. **(b)** A child who neither has been expected to concentrate nor appreciated for doing so is likely to be slow in acquiring the capacity for attention. Under the age of 5 years, attention is stimulus bound, and between 5 and 7 years of age, a shift occurs in a child's ability to attend as attention comes under the control of inner logical processes. Between 3 and 8 years of age, measures of sustained attention, reaction time, and motor inhibition have shown a strong social class effect, and these factors have improved exponentially around the same period, especially between ages 4 and 6 years. *(Ref. 3, pp. 229–230)*

50. **(b)** Difficulties and delays at an early stage of language development can keep a child behind, which produces an increased risk for psychopathology and learning difficulties. No data or evidence support the causal relationship between language development and low intelligence. *(Ref. 3, p. 250)*

51. **(c)** Compared to boys, girls' genital self-stimulation (masturbation) tends to begin later, is less constant, and shows less intentional arousal. Masturbation may occur without pleasure. Girls use more indirect techniques and experience more overt disturbance and anxiety about masturbation than boys. *(Ref. 3, pp. 278–279)*

52. **(c)** Studies show fathers are less involved in care-taking activities than mothers, but more involved in playing with their children in more stimulating and unconventional ways. Active involvement of fathers not only facilitates the development of gender identity and role, but also more likely results in more masculine sons and more feminine daughters. Absence of a father's involvement produces opposite and negative effects on a child's sexual development. *(Ref. 3, p. 280)*

53. **(d)** By 1 to 2 years of age, normal children have established a core gender identity (i.e., a sense of being male or female). By 2.5 years of age, they can categorize men and women by sex. Transsexualism is a disorder of gender identity (gender identity disorder) characterized by the transsexual individual's belief that she or he belongs to the opposite sex. Homosexuality involves the erotic attraction between individuals of the same sex, who view this attraction as congruous with their biologic sex. Gender identity is usually stable throughout one's lifetime, with reported instances where a few people changed their identity with success. *(Ref. 1, p. 813; Ref. 3, p. 275)*

54. **(e)** There are significant physical, cognitive, and psychological changes in normal adolescent development. Girls start puberty around age 9 to 11 years—approximately 2 years earlier than boys. Along with a remodeling process (pruning) of cortical synapses and neurobiological changes, adolescents make dramatic growth in cognition with a greater ability in abstract thinking; most reach Piaget's formal operational stage. They are more aware of their body image, with some gender differences. Girls are more likely than boys to perceive themselves as overweight and more girls than boys attempt to lose weight. While there are conflicts in families with adolescents, studies show an association between authoritative parenting and better outcomes for adolescents. *(Ref. 3, pp. 333–336)*

55. **(e)** Menstruation can be delayed or stopped by maintaining a low fat-to-muscle ratio as happens with excessive exercise and dieting. Cessation of menses may also occur with extreme stress. Alteration in normal endocrine functioning, such as hypothalamic hypogonadism, may result in amenorrhea. *(Ref. 3, pp. 108–110, 693–695)*

56. (d) Homosexual contacts are more frequent in early adolescence, some of which are transient and do not necessarily lead to sexual orientation as gay/lesbian or homosexual. Strong evidence exists to support genetic influences in the establishment of homosexuality based on twin studies. Localized neurosteroids affect brain and subsequently sexual orientation. Interestingly, some studies show that sons born later in order are more likely to be homosexual. *(Ref. 3, pp. 275–277, 282)*

57. (c) Recent studies show that not all adolescents are severely emotionally disturbed, and 80% of them do not experience any turmoil. Even though only a minority develops major affective disorders, some studies show one third of adolescents experience depression. The CDC high school survey data indicated relatively high rates of sadness and hopelessness, and of suicidal ideation. Some gender differences were noticed and girls tended to experience more mood symptoms than boys. As a group, adolescents demonstrated more variations in their mood states than adults. *(Ref. 3, pp. 339–340)*

58. (a) A recent longitudinal study found that reaching Tanner stage III was associated with increasing depression in girls. Both male and female hormonal levels were also associated with the severity of depression. A 2000 study by Spear hypothesized that adolescents' novelty seeking can be a compensatory mechanism due to the imbalance of dopamine regulation in the prefrontal cortex. Adolescents are accident prone and engage in more risk-taking behavior, which can be a serious source of morbidity and mortality. To distinguish late adolescence and early adulthood from other periods of life, Arnett (2000) proposed a term "emerging adulthood" to categorize the time from the late teens through the twenties. *(Ref. 3, pp. 340–341)*

59. (d) Different family structures (whether they are nuclear families, adoptive families, single-mother families, or foster families) all encounter the same developmental tasks. Adolescents become more autonomous. Different boundaries compared to those used in families with younger children are developed to deal with the new family dynamics and the conflicts between independence and dependence. Parents, as well as teenagers, experience significant stress to accommodate the new homeostasis in the family. Interestingly, a study showed adolescents with bulimia rated their fathers as less affectionate and controlling than did their siblings without bulimia. Having different biological preparation time, adoptive families can still sometimes follow a psychological pathway similar to that of nuclear families. *(Ref. 3, p. 291)*

60. (d) Due to limited cognitive ability, very young children do not understand the irreversibility of death; rather, they may perceive death as abandonment, and blame their own misbehavior, which can result in their feelings of guilt, sadness, and anger. School-age children with increased cognitive and emotional maturity start to grasp the concept of death and its irreversible and inevitable nature. *(Ref. 1, p. 39)*

61. (e) While depressed and anxious children are likely to misperceive threats and external demands, children with high impulsivity and hyperactivity tend to show deficits in information processing, lack of self-control, and failure in verbal

mediation. According to Beck, everyone possesses a unique way to see his or her own self, others, and the world, which he referred to as a schema through which people make their own interpretations of the world. Cognitive therapists believe particular schema can be the source of a clinical disorder. Cognitive–behavioral therapy is integration of a cognitive approach with a behavioral approach that focuses more on observable behavior and environmental stressors. This therapy can help children and adolescents build positive cognitive structures that influence their future life. *(Ref. 3, pp. 157–158)*

62. (d) In the United States, the individual is encouraged to become physically and verbally assertive, whereas in Japan, the individual is encouraged to become physically and verbally restrained. These values are related to child-rearing practices. American infants are raised more independently than Asian infants. In the United States, White children have been shown to have a stronger internal locus of control than Black children, a finding explained by majority/minority status. Native American children are raised to value allegiance to the family and community more highly than allegiance to the self. Asian mothers believe in their children's academic ability more than mothers born in the United States. Children in Asian countries are expected to work hard for academic achievements. *(Ref. 3, pp. 494–495)*

63. (b) Serotonin is produced from hydroxylation and decarboxylation of the amino acid tryptophan. The rate-limiting step is the hydroxylation of tryptophan to form 5-hydroxytryptophan, catalyzed by the enzyme tryptophan hydroxylase. Tyrosine hydroxylase, on the other hand, is the rate-limiting enzyme for the synthesis of dopamine and norepinephrine. *(Ref. 3, pp. 47–49)*

64. (d) The serotonin metabolite is 5-HIAA. Metabolites of neurotransmitters can be found in cerebrospinal fluid, blood, and urine. Studies measuring metabolites of neurotransmitter ontogeny have helped us understand neurochemistry of normal development. Monoamine oxidase and COMT are two main enzymes responsible for the metabolism of many neurotransmitters. The metabolites of norepinephrine are MHPG and VMA. The metabolites of dopamine are HVA and DOPAC. *(Ref. 3, pp. 49–52)*

65. (d) Cholinergic deficit can cause Alzheimer's disease. Cholinergic neurons in the forebrain can project to different locations, including the entire cortex, hippocampus, and amygdala. Through the projections to these areas, acetylcholine modulates attention, novelty seeking, and memory. *(Ref. 3, pp. 946)*

66. (b) Gabaergic interneurons (short-ranging neurons) can be found in the cortex, thalamus, striatum, cerebellum, and spinal cord; long-range neurons can be found in the basal ganglia, septum, and substantia nigra. Gabaergic neurons in the cortex and thalamus are crucial for inhibiting the excitatory neurons. This inhibition is believed to be of benefit to the treatment of anxiety disorders, insomnia, and agitation. *(Ref. 3, pp. 947–948)*

67. (e) Glutamatergic neurons can be located in different areas throughout the brain, affecting brain functions in many ways by binding to NMDA, AMPA, and Kainate receptors. Binding of glutamate to glutamatergic neurons and NMDA receptors in the hippocampus is crucial in the formation of memory resulting from the creation of long-term potentiation. *(Ref. 3, p. 948)*

Matching

68. (b) The developmental task of the very young infant is to achieve adaptation to the outside world.

69. (a) Between 1.5 and 3 years of age, children make a shift from a passive to an active position, which is due in large part to neuromuscular maturation and the ability to think and communicate.

70. (d) During the school-age period of development, children move toward greater separation, independence, and autonomy while, at the same time, being demanding, intrusive, and negative.

71. (c) During adolescence, tasks include defining oneself, achieving separation from the family, developing love relationships outside the family, and achieving mastery over impulses and bodily capacities. *(Questions 68–71: Ref. 1, pp. 35–37)*

72. (c); 73. (b); 74. (d); 75. (a) In addition to the foregoing relationships, Piaget's sensorimotor stage correlates with Freud's oral stage, his preoperational stage correlates with Freud's anal and phallic stages, his concrete operational stage correlates with Freud's latency stage, and his formal operational stage correlates with Freud's adolescence stage. *(Ref. 1, pp. 20, 31–32, 36)*

76. (b) The frontal lobes are most concerned with motor and executive functions, such as speaking, organizing, and planning complex activities. Defects lead to aphasias, certain kinds of apraxias, and deficits of attention and in the planning and execution of complex behavior.

77. (d) The temporal lobes have emotional and memory functions, and sensory functions associated with visceral sensations, olfaction, hearing, and speech. Defects can result in negative symptoms, amnesias, and emotional disturbances of blandness or poor emotional regulation.

78. (a) The basal ganglia modulate motor and some autonomic functions are involved in intellectual functions, especially the maintenance of attention.

79. (c) The reticular system contains homeostatic, postural, activating (noradrenergic), and incoming information-modulating (serotonergic and dopaminergic) sections. *(Questions 76–79: Ref. 3, pp. 125–127)*

80. (b) John Bowlby utilized developmental psychology and evolutionary biology to propose that infant–mother attachment not only is a result of the mother's association with the gratification of urges, but also is due to species-typical behaviors that evolved to promote infant survival.

81. (c) Assimilation and accommodation were terms used by Piaget to describe the way in which an organism creates and adapts to new knowledge.

82. (a) Winnicott used the term "transitional object" to describe the first "not-me" object, such as a soft blanket or a cuddly toy to be used for comfort when the mother is unavailable to provide comforting.

83. (e) Klein postulated a rich inner life of the infant with many sexual and aggressive fantasies. Reparation was a term she used to refer to the return to the mother after she became the fantasized object of the infant's attacks for withholding gratification.

84. (f) In their New York Longitudinal Study, Chess and Thomas utilized the terms "goodness of fit" and "poorness of fit" to describe the match of the infant's temperament with the environment/caregivers.

85. (d) Anna Freud strove to create a developmental theory based on the unfolding of sexual and aggressive urges in relationship to the child's parents and environment. *(Questions 80–85: Ref. 3, pp. 164–166, 174, 207–208, 222, 258, 307, 993)*

86. (c) Denial is an unconscious mechanism that allows the adolescent to avoid awareness of thoughts, feelings, wishes, needs, or external reality factors that are consciously intolerable.

87. (f) (projection of guilt) Projection is the unconscious mechanism whereby an unacceptable impulse, feeling, or idea is attributed to the external world.

88. (j) Splitting occurs when the adolescent unconsciously views people or events as being at one extreme or the other.

89. (n) Acting out takes place when unconscious emotional conflicts or feelings are expressed in an arena that is different from the one in which they arose. Generally, acting out is a feeling expressed in actions rather than in words.

90. (d) Regression is a partial or symbolic return to more infantile patterns of reacting or thinking.

91. (k) Counterphobia is seeking out experiences that are consciously or unconsciously feared.

92. (o) Identification occurs when a person unconsciously patterns himself or herself after some other person. (Role modeling or imitation is similar to identification, but is a conscious process.)

93. (e) Reaction formation unconsciously transforms unacceptable feelings, ideas, or impulses into their opposites.

94. (a) Repression (unconscious) and suppression (conscious) occur when unacceptable thoughts, wishes, or impulses that would produce anxiety are pushed out of awareness.

95. (b) Displacement takes place when emotions, ideas, or wishes are transferred from their original source or target to a more acceptable substitute.

96. (i) Isolation of affect is the separation of ideas or events from the feelings associated with them.

97. (m) Rationalization uses reasoning and "rational" explanations, which may or may not be valid, to explain away unconscious conflicts and motivations.

98. (h) Intellectualization controls affects and impulse by analyzing through excessive thought without experiencing the feeling.

99. **(p)** Sublimation unconsciously replaces an unacceptable feeling with a course of action that is personally and socially acceptable.

100. **(l)** Humor is used defensively to relieve anxiety caused by the discrepancies between what one wishes for himself or herself and what actually happens.

101. **(g)** Altruism is a seemingly unselfish interest in the welfare of others. *(Questions 86–101: Ref. 3, pp. 199, 977; Ref. 4, pp. 807–813)*

102. **(c)** Most noradrenergic neurons in the brain arise from the locus ceruleus and are thought to play a role in anxiety and panic disorders.

103. **(a)** Dopamine is the major neurotransmitter in the pigmented substantia nigra that degenerates in Parkinson's disease.

104. **(b)** The midline raphe nuclei contain serotonin, which is important in sleep and some types of depression. *(Questions 102–104: Ref. 3, pp. 47–50, 125–127)*

2

DEVELOPMENTAL DISORDERS

QUESTIONS

Directions: Select the best response for each of the questions 1–30.

1. Which one of the following neurotransmitter systems shows the greatest alteration in autism?
   a. Norepinephrine
   b. Dopamine
   c. Acetylcholine
   d. Serotonin
   e. Epinephrine

2. Which of the following percentages is an accurate estimate of the prevalence of mental retardation in the general population?
   a. 0.25%
   b. 0.50%
   c. 1%
   d. 2%
   e. 3%

3. Neural tube defects are associated with all of the following disorders *except:*
   a. Hydrocephalus
   b. Arnold–Chiari II malformation
   c. Trisomy 18 syndrome
   d. Spina bifida
   e. Neural tube closure defect by 18 to 28 days of gestation

4. *The Diagnostic and Statistical Manual of Mental Disorders* (Fourth Edition) Text Revision (DSM-IV-TR) diagnostic criteria for autistic disorder lists four general categories in which particular symptoms should be present. Which of the following categories is *not* among the DSM-IV-TR diagnostic criteria?
   a. Impairment in intellectual functioning
   b. Impairment in reciprocal interaction
   c. Impairment in verbal and nonverbal communication
   d. Markedly restricted repertoire of activities and interests
   e. Onset before 36 months of age

5. Which of the following statements regarding the etiology of autism is *not* an accurate reflection of the current state of knowledge?
   a. Autism does not seem to have a hereditary component.
   b. Congenital factors are important in the etiology of autism.
   c. An immunity defect may play a role in the development of autism.
   d. Neurologic abnormalities are frequently found in autistic individuals.
   e. Cerebellar hypoplasia is found in some autistic individuals.

6. Which one of the following factors is the *most* consistently related to the outcome of autism?
   a. Amount of time spent in school
   b. Rating of social behavior
   c. Comorbid neuropsychiatric disorders
   d. Presence or absence of speech
   e. Rating of social maturity

7. Individuals with Asperger's syndrome usually demonstrate all of the following *except:*
   a. Curiosity about the environment
   b. Impairments in reciprocal social interactions
   c. Impaired cognitive and language development
   d. Restricted and repetitive behaviors
   e. Normal self-help skills and adaptive behavior

8. Rett's syndrome is characterized by all of the following *except:*
   a. Apparently normal prenatal and perinatal growth and development
   b. Deceleration of head growth, development of hypotonia, and loss of interest in play activity
   c. "Autistic features"
   d. Greater prevalence in boys
   e. Diagnosis tentative until 2 to 5 years of age

9. Childhood disintegrative disorder is characterized by all of the following *except:*
   a. Apparently normal development up to the age of at least 2 years
   b. Severe lower motor neuron and basal ganglia dysfunction
   c. A definite loss of previously acquired social, language, and/or motor skills at about the time of onset of the disorder
   d. Abnormal social functioning
   e. An association with severe mental retardation

10. Which of the following learning and communication disorders is considered the *most* socially disabling and severe?
    a. Mathematics disorder
    b. Reading disorder
    c. Phonological disorder
    d. Stuttering
    e. Mixed receptive–expressive language disorder

11. Which of the following are *least* likely to have co-occurring autism?
    a. Down's syndrome
    b. Angelman's syndrome
    c. Tuberous sclerosis
    d. Fragile X syndrome
    e. Phenylketonuria (PKU)

12. All of the following are common pharmacotherapy mistakes for treating people with mental retardation *except:*

a. Treatment of single nonspecific symptom with lack of diagnostic understanding

b. Continuation of treatment without effectiveness

c. Consideration of potential different side effects from the medicines

d. Pharmacotherapy alone without other psychosocial interventions

e. Substitution of education and training with psychotropic medications

13. Mental retardation is defined by all of the following *except:*

a. Low IQ

b. Onset before the age of 18

c. Observable deficits in adaptive behaviors

d. Deficits in more than one cognitive process

e. Clinical judgment made on infant's or untestable children's intellectual functioning

14. All of the following conditions/disorders are more prevalent in people with mental retardation *except:*

a. Autism

b. Pica

c. Stuttering

d. Attention-deficit hyperactivity disorder (ADHD)

e. Rumination

15. The etiology of mental retardation can be categorized into three groups: (1) errors in morphogenesis of central nervous system (CNS); (2) errors related to the intrinsic biological environment; (3) extrinsic factors. All of the following conditions/syndromes are due to CNS malformations that commonly lead to mental retardation *except:*

a. Prader–Willi syndrome

b. Pena–Shokeir syndrome

c. Cerebral palsy

d. Down's syndrome

e. Myelodysplasia (spina bifida)

16. Babies and young children having an uncomplicated mental retardation are *most* likely to show all of the following behaviors as early symptoms of retardation *except:*

a. Delayed attachment behaviors

b. Less activity

c. Delayed development of verbal communication

d. Less compliance

e. Less readiness to respond to their parents

17. Which of the following genetic variations is strongly associated with Rett's disorder?

a. Mutation of MECP2 gene

b. Mutation of FMR1 gene

c. Deletion of an elastin gene

d. Deletion of chromosome 15p11q13

e. Trisomy 21

18. All of the following statements regarding intelligence in autistic children are correct *except:*

a. Studies show most autistic children are retarded.

b. Those with low IQ are more likely to develop seizures.

c. Those with low IQ are more likely to show deviant social responses.

d. Low IQ is associated with poorer prognosis.

e. Low IQ is usually due to low motivation of the autistic subjects.

19. Asperger's syndrome is *least* likely to have which of the following features?

a. Lack of social intuition

b. Normal intelligence

c. Obsessive preoccupation or circumscribed interests

d. The presence of hallucinations and delusions

e. No significant delay in language

20. Symptoms of mental disorders often associated with autistic disorder include all of the following *except:*

a. Obsessive–compulsive behaviors and tics

b. Hallucinations and delusions

c. Inattention and hyperactivity

d. Irritability and other mood symptoms

e. Anxiety

21. All of the following statements regarding the epidemiology of autism accurately reflect the state of current knowledge *except:*

a. The prevalence of autism is between 2 and 6 instances per 1000 Americans.

b. Recent studies show generally higher prevalence rates than in the past.

c. Families of autistic individuals are primarily upper class.

d. Rates of the disorder are four to five times higher in males than in females.

e. Girls tend to suffer a greater degree of morbidity.

22. In the DSM-IV-TR, pervasive developmental disorder not otherwise specified (PDDNOS) is characterized by all of the following statements *except:*

a. It includes those individuals who share many, although not all, of the features of infantile autism.

b. It is more common than autistic disorder.

c. It includes persons with less severe symptoms of socialization, communication, and repetitive activities than does autistic disorder.

d. It represents a narrow, homogeneous group of characteristics.

e. In unstructured description tasks, children with PDDNOS use fewer inner, psychological concepts as descriptors than typically developing children.

23. The assessment of language function involves all of the following *except:*

a. Phonation

b. Comprehension
c. Syntax and morphology
d. Semantics
e. Outer language

24. Learning disorders are accurately characterized by all of the following statements *except:*
    a. 75% of children with learning disorders have significant social skills deficits.
    b. Many individuals (10 to 25%) with conduct disorder, oppositional defiant disorder, attention-deficit hyperactivity disorder, major depressive disorder, or dysthymic disorder also have learning disorders.
    c. The etiology may include a variety of neurocognitive defects.
    d. Approximately 15% of students in public schools in the United States have a learning disorder.
    e. Based on DSM and the Individuals with Disabilities Education Act of 2004 (IDEA), the discrepancy model is used for diagnostic purposes.

25. Selective mutism is characterized by all of the following statements *except:*
    a. Subjects often refuse to speak outside the home.
    b. The onset is usually between 3 and 8 years of age.
    c. Social environment factors can contribute to the development of the disorder.
    d. There is a lack of adequate knowledge of the language.
    e. There is a strong association with social phobia.

26. All of the following statements regarding mild mental retardation (MR) are accurate *except:*
    a. The IQ ranges from 50 to 55 to approximately 70.
    b. Individuals with mild MR may acquire academic skills up to the sixth grade.
    c. Mild MR represents about 85% of the retarded population.
    d. Individuals with mild MR may need supervision and assistance.
    e. Most individuals with mild retardation need to live in highly structured settings.

27. All of the following statements concerning individuals with Fragile X syndrome are accurate reflections of current knowledge *except:*
    a. Females are more likely to present with more variable intellectual functioning.
    b. Fragile X syndrome is one of the leading etiologies of inherited mental retardation.
    c. Males are more likely to present difficulties with math, anxiety, and attention deficit.
    d. Males are more likely to present with impairments of visuospatial and memory function.

e. Fragile X syndrome results from disruption of the expression of the fragile X gene.

28. According to the Individuals with Disabilities Education Act of 2004 (IDEA), younger children (age 3 to 9 years) with disabilities who are eligible for special education can also receive all of the following related services *except:*
    a. Transportation
    b. Developmental, corrective, and other supportive services
    c. Speech–language, audiological, and counseling services
    d. Physical and occupational therapies
    e. Medical treatments

29. Which one of the following tests was designed to measure adaptive functioning?
    a. Leiter International Performance Scale, Revised
    b. Vineland Adaptive Behavior Scale
    c. Stanford–Binet
    d. Kaufman Assessment Battery for Children (K-ABC)
    e. Rorschach Inkblot

30. All of the following statements are correct regarding learning disorders, motor skill disorders, and communication disorders *except:*
    a. They are commonly comorbid with other psychiatric disorders.
    b. Evidence suggests a significant association between communication disorders and learning disorders.
    c. They have a strong association with ADHD based on epidemiological studies.
    d. Deficits in intellectual functioning are considered as diagnostic features.
    e. Boys have higher prevalence rates for learning disorders and communication disorders than girls.

Matching

31–34. For each of the syndromes usually associated with mental retardation listed, select from the following one description that fits it best:
    a. Diet prevents mental retardation
    b. Obesity
    c. Microcephaly and medial epicanthal folds
    d. Motor and cognitive deterioration

31. Prader–Willi syndrome
32. Down's syndrome
33. Phenylketonuria
34. Niemann–Pick disease

ANSWERS AND EXPLANATIONS

1. **(d)** The majority of the studies of 5-hydroxytryptamine (5-HT) (serotonin) reveal hyperserotonemia in autism. Based on measurements of cerebrospinal-fluid 3-methoxy-4-hydroxyphenyl-glycol (MHPG) and studies of plasma or urine norepinephrine, MHPG, and vanily mandelic acid, one can tentatively conclude that noradrenergic functioning is not greatly altered in autism. Central dopamine functioning, to the extent it can be measured by current measures, is normal in autism. *(Ref. 1, pp. 291–292; Ref. 3, pp. 53–55, 101)*

2. **(c)** It is estimated that 1% of the general population would be diagnosed as mentally retarded. The highest prevalence is in the 10- to 20-year-old age group, probably reflecting the fact that mild mental retardation may become more obvious during school age. *(Ref. 1, p. 224; Ref. 4, p. 46)*

3. **(c)** Hydrocephalus, Arnold–Chiari II syndrome, and spina bifida are all the result of early abnormal formation of the neural tube *in utero*. Trisomy 18 syndrome is associated with a chromosomal anomaly. It results in profound retardation and has a low survival rate. *(Ref. 1, p. 227)*

4. **(a)** All of the categories listed are in the criteria except impairment in intellectual functioning, although 75% of children with autistic disorder function at a retarded level. The DSM-III-R did not have the criterion of age of onset of abnormal functioning prior to 3 years. However, DSM-IV-TR does. *(Ref. 4, p. 75)*

5. **(a)** Based on a review of studies, autism has a hereditary component and perinatal complications are contributory in some cases. Depressed immune function, autoimmune mechanisms, or faulty immune regulation may be associated with the etiology of autism. Neurologic abnormalities are reported in 30 to 75% of autistic individuals. *(Ref. 1, pp. 275–281; Ref. 3, pp. 591–592)*

6. **(d)** There are three factors that are more consistently associated with the outcome of autism, including: (1) the presence or absence of speech; (2) IQ; and (3) the severity of the disorder. Less robust factors are: (1) amount of time spent in school; (2) rating of social maturity; (3) rating of social behavior; (4) achievement of developmental milestones; and (5) comorbid neuropsychiatric disorders. More controversial factors include sex, brain dysfunction or damage, and so on. *(Ref. 1, p. 296)*

7. **(c)** Individuals with Asperger's syndrome do not have a clinically significant general delay in language or cognitive development. While they are interested in human relationships, they are unable to carry through on social interactions with sufficient success to make relationships easy. As individuals with autism, they have restricted, repetitive, and stereotyped patterns of behavior, interests, and activities. *(Ref. 1, pp. 318–320; Ref. 4, pp. 80–84)*

8. **(d)** Rett's syndrome is thought to be a genetically determined neurodegenerative disorder in which growth and development are normal during the first 5 months up to 18 months, but then there is developmental regression between 5 months and 48 months, followed by stereotypic hand movements, severely impaired expressive and receptive language, severe psychomotor retardation, and social withdrawal. The disorder has been reported only in females. *(Ref. 1, pp. 325–328; Ref. 4, pp. 76–77)*

9. **(b)** Children with childhood disintegrative disorder have normal age-appropriate skills in communication, social relationships, play, and adaptive behavior at the age of 2 years. There is a definite loss of previously acquired skills at about the time of onset of the disorder. Abnormal social functioning resembling autism occurs. It is distinguished from Rett's syndrome as only Rett's is marked by the severe, lower motor neuron and basal ganglia dysfunction. *(Ref. 1, pp. 334–338; Ref. 4, pp. 77–79)*

10. **(e)** Children with mixed receptive–expressive language disorders show deficits in expression as well as in comprehension of language. As a result, it is the most disabling and severe of the disorders listed. *(Ref. 1, p. 369)*

11. **(a)** Autism is found less frequently associated with Down's syndrome than in the general population. It is observed more commonly in all of the other syndromes listed. However, these associations are by no means invariable. *(Ref. 3, p. 591; Ref. 4, p. 72)*

12. **(c)** The usual principles of psychopharmacologic management apply equally well to retarded and nonretarded individuals, without evidence to suggest different mechanisms of drug action or effectiveness in people with mental retardation. However, the effectiveness of medicines may differ among various syndromes associated with mental retardation. People with mental retardation are more susceptible to side effects. The diagnostic assessment may require additional attention beyond simply diagnosing retardation, since patients may have other coexisting disorders and their communication skills may be less developed. *(Ref. 1, pp. 253–254)*

13. **(d)** Mental retardation is defined in the DSM-IV-TR as an IQ of approximately 70 or below, impairments in adaptive functioning, and onset before 18 years of age. For infants, clinical judgment can be used to determine the intellectual functioning. While there may be deficits in one or more cognitive processes, the number of deficits is not a diagnostic consideration. *(Ref. 1, pp. 222–224; Ref. 4, pp. 41–44)*

14. **(d)** Based on limited prevalence data on the epidemiology of psychopathology in people with mental retardation, it is generally agreed that youth with mental retardation are at higher risk for developing other mental disorders. However, the prevalence of ADHD seems to be similar in the general population compared to the mentally retarded population. Some conditions/disorders occur at higher rates in youth with mental retardation, including pica, rumination, stuttering, and autism. *(Ref. 1, pp. 241–242, 246; Ref. 2, pp. 181–182)*

15. (c) The syndromes listed are examples of CNS malformations that can result in mental retardation, except for cerebral palsy, which is a developmental disorder of motor function and of cerebral or cerebellar origin. People with cerebral palsy do not necessarily experience cognitive impairment or mental retardation. Errors of morphogenesis include malformation syndromes, *in utero* neurologic disease, and injury to the central nervous system. Both inborn errors of metabolism and noninborn errors of metabolism, such as those resulting from hypoglycemia secondary to sepsis or cerebral edema secondary to hepatic encephalopathy, are etiologic, as are such extrinsic influences as trauma, hypoxia, and poisoning. *(Ref. 1, pp. 225–231)*

16. (d) Retarded infants demonstrate fewer attachment behaviors and respond less readily to their parents, appear less active, are less interactive vocally, and tend to be more compliant as compared with nonretarded infants of the same mental or chronological age. *(Ref. 1, pp. 238–239)*

17. (a) Recent studies show that 35 to 100% of patients with typical Rett's disorder carry a mutation in the encoding region of the X-linked MECP2 gene, which has been considered as the genetic etiology of Rett's disorder. Mutation of the FMR1 gene, deletion of an elastin gene, deletion of chromosome 15p11q13, and Trisomy 21 are some possible genetic etiologies of fragile X syndrome, Williams syndrome, Angelman's syndrome, and Down's syndrome, respectively. *(Ref. 1, pp. 226–228; 328–329)*

18. (e) Studies show low IQ testing scores are not associated with poor motivation of children with autism being tested. It has been reported that most autistic children (40 to 60%) have an IQ below 50 and some (20 to 30%) have an IQ of 70 or higher. During the standard testing, autistic children do better on performance subtests requiring visual–spatial skills (such as block design) or immediate memory, and worse on tasks demanding symbolic or abstract thought and sequential logic. Epilepsy is more prevalent in autistic children with low IQ and both seizure and low IQ are associated with a poorer prognosis. *(Ref. 1, pp. 266–267)*

19. (d) The main features of Asperger's syndrome are a lack of social intuition, leading to naïve and tactless behavior and difficulty with social relationships; normal intelligence without a significant delay in language development, but with poor coordination and visual–spatial perception; and obsessive preoccupation or circumscribed interest patterns. Hallucinations and delusions are not common features of Asperger's syndrome. *(Ref. 1, pp. 318–319; Ref. 4, pp. 80–84)*

20. (b) More highly functioning autistic children demonstrate ritualistic, repetitive, and compulsive behaviors. They also demonstrate tics from time to time. However, autistic individuals rarely have hallucinations or delusions. Other highly comorbid psychiatric symptoms may include poor attention/concentration and hyperactivity, anxiety, and mood symptoms. *(Ref. 1, pp. 268–269)*

21. (c) In contrast to earlier biased studies, newer data show autistic individuals are found in all socioeconomic classes. Epidemiological studies from different countries show prevalence rates of autism fall between 0.0015 and 0.34%. There is a trend toward increased prevalence rates of autism since the early 1980s. Based on prevalence statistics from the National Institutes of Health (2004), the 2000 U.S. Census figure of 280 million Americans, and the Centers for Disease Control and Prevention (2001), 1 out of 166 births is diagnosed with autism, and the autism prevalence rate is 2 to 6 per 1000. Studies also demonstrate ratios of four to five autistic boys to one autistic girl, and autistic girls tend to suffer a greater degree of morbidity and a higher rate of comorbid seizures. *(Ref. 1, pp. 273–274; Ref. 3, p. 589; Ref. 4, p. 73)*

22. (d) According to DSM-IV-TR, PDDNOS can be diagnosed when there is severe and pervasive impairment in development in the same core domains (social interaction; communications; restricted, repetitive, and stereotyped patterns of behaviors) as the impairment seen in autism, but the criteria are not met for a specific PDD or other related disorders. PDDNOS, a more common condition than autism, represents a more heterogeneous (not homogenous) group of conditions that share autistic-like features. Based on some studies, compared to normal children, children with PPDNOS may have poor motor development, confused and bizarre thinking, anxiety and perseveration, and their social impairment may manifest as a tenuous, brittle, and shallow manner of relating to others. In completing emotional role-taking tasks, children with PDDNOS use fewer inner, psychological characteristics. *(Ref. 1, pp. 338–339; Ref. 4, p. 84)*

23. (e) In psychiatric assessment for language, inner (not outer) language, comprehension, production, and pragmatics are the specific areas clinicians should focus on. Phonation refers to voice quality, including pitch, volume, intonation, and prosody. Morphology refers to the use of inflectional endings and functional words. Syntax refers to word order, use of pronouns, and verb tense. Semantics refers to the range of vocabulary. *(Ref. 1, pp. 365–366)*

24. (d) Approximately 5% (not 15%) of students in public schools in the United States have a learning disorder. It is quite common for children who ultimately are diagnosed as learning disabled to present initially with emotional or behavioral problems. Poor self-esteem, anxiety, alienation, and/or rebellion can be the result of learning disability. Learning-disabled children may have difficulty in developing strategies for organizing, prioritizing, rehearsing, or presenting information. A majority (75%) of children with learning disorders show significant social skills deficits. Even though the discrepancy model was not empirically validated, it is still used for diagnosing learning disorders based on DSM and IDEA. *(Ref. 1, pp. 352–359; Ref. 4, pp. 48–51)*

25. (d) Selective mutism is most commonly manifested by a refusal to speak outside the home despite often speaking normally within the home. There is often a history of family isolation, a shy or uncommunicative parent, a broken family, and an overly strong attachment to the mother. The onset of selective mutism can be insidious and as early as approximately age 3 years, but often the diagnosis is made between 3 and 8 years of age. Some authors believe selective mutism is associated with social phobia and can be viewed as a symptom of it rather than as a separate phenomenon. Children with selective mutism may have certain communication disorders, but they usually have adequate knowledge of the language that they speak. *(Ref. 1, pp. 596–598; Ref. 4, pp. 125–127)*

26. **(e)** Most individuals with mild retardation make it to the sixth grade and are able to live in community residences. In contrast, those with moderate mental retardation reach only the second grade in school, and those with severe mental retardation need to live in highly structured settings. However, mildly retarded individuals may need supervision, assistance, and guidance especially when under stress. *(Ref. 4, pp. 42–43)*

27. **(c)** Fragile X syndrome is caused by the disruption of the expression of the fragile X gene (FMR1) secondary to its mutation. This mutation leads to a lower level of production of the fragile X mental retardation protein (FMRP), which results in the interference of normal brain development and the unique phenotypes of this syndrome. Fragile X syndrome is one the most common causes of inherited mental retardation, occurring in 0.025 to 0.05% of live births in both genders. However, it may manifest differently in certain aspects, mainly because it is an X-linked disorder. In girls, there are more difficulties with math, anxiety, and inattention, with more variable intellectual functioning, whereas in boys there are more difficulties with visuospatial and memory function, mental retardation, and hyperactivity. Both girls and boys can present with poor social communication skills. *(Ref. 3, pp. 140–141)*

28. **(e)** Special education programs are becoming more sophisticated in treating developmentally disabled children and their families. The right to a free appropriate public education in the least restrictive environment is guaranteed by a federal law—the 1975 Education for All Handicapped Children Act (EAHCA, also known as Public Law 94-142). EAHCA was revised in 1991 and became IDEA. IDEA grants states the option of extending special education and related services to children below age 9. All listed services are under the category of "related services," except for medical treatments (only diagnostic and evaluative service is covered, not medical treatments). *(Ref. 3, pp. 1370–1371; the Individuals with Disabilities Education Act of 2004, Public Law 108-446, 108th Congress)*

29. **(b)** In addition to Scales of Independent Behavior (DLM Teaching Resources), the Vineland Adaptive Behavior Scale is designed to measure adaptive functioning or behavior. The Wechsler Intelligence Scale for Children, K-ABC, and the Stanford–Binet are all standardized intelligence tests but are not specifically designed to measure adaptive functioning. The Leiter International Performance Scale, Revised, is also a test to measure intellectual ability, especially for nonverbal individuals. The Rorschach Inkblot, considered as a projective test, is not designed to measure adaptive functioning. *(Ref. 3, pp. 558–559)*

30. **(d)** Deficient intellectual functioning is not a diagnostic feature. Presence of cognitive impairments and sensory deficits is allowed, but the emphasis is on the discrepancy between the achievement and the degree of those deficits/impairments. Based on DSM-IV-TR, motor skill disorder is categorized together with learning disorders and communication disorders. Learning disorders include reading disorder, mathematics disorder, disorder of written expression, and learning disorder, not otherwise specified (NOS). Communication disorders (also called language disorders) include expressive language disorder, mixed receptive–expressive language disorder, phonological disorder, and communication disorder, NOS. All the other statements are correct. *(Ref. 1, pp. 351–353)*

Matching

31. **(b)** Prader–Willi syndrome, which is associated with the deletion of q11-q13 on chromosome 15 in more than 70% of cases, is characterized by hypotonia, obesity, small hands and feet, hyperphagia, narrow forehead, downward-slanted palpebral fissures, an IQ between 20 and 80, and frequent behavioral problems.

32. **(c)** Down's syndrome, or Trisomy 21, is characterized by microcephaly, hypotonia, medial epicanthal folds, small ears, and an IQ range of 25 to 50, manifesting early symptomatology of Alzheimer's disease.

33. **(a)** Phenylketonuria is a disorder of amino-acid metabolism in which the infant is normal at birth, but progresses to vomiting and irritability, and then to developmental delay, seizures, microcephaly, and spasticity. A phenylalanine-restricted diet prevents mental retardation, and prenatal diagnosis is possible.

34. **(d)** Niemann–Pick disease is due to a disorder in sphingomyelinase lipid metabolism that results in hepatosplenomegaly, cherry-red macula, motor and cognitive deterioration after normal milestones, and possible profound mental retardation. *(Ref. 1, pp. 225–230)*

3

SCHIZOPHRENIA SPECTRUM DISORDERS AND AFFECTIVE DISORDERS

QUESTIONS

Directions: Select the best response for each of the questions 1–35.

1. The DSM-IV-TR criteria for the diagnosis of schizophrenia in children and adolescents is the same as in adults *except for:*

   a. Presence of hallucinations
   b. Duration of at least 6 months
   c. Functioning below the highest level previously achieved
   d. Presence of delusions
   e. Deficient social relations

2. Typically, the onset of schizophrenia usually occurs in which of the following age groups?

   a. Preschool-age children
   b. Latency-age children
   c. Early teens
   d. Late teens to the mid-30s
   e. Late 30s

3. All of the following statements regarding childhood schizophrenia are true *except:*

   a. The first prominent premorbid signs of dysfunction are withdrawal and impairments in adaptive social behavior.
   b. Affective disturbance is common.
   c. Catatonic symptoms are common.
   d. A majority of patients experience hallucinations.
   e. Most patients have low average to average range of intellectual functioning.

4. All of the following statements regarding the age of onset of schizophrenia are accurate according to the current literature *except:*

   a. It seldom becomes manifest before 5 years of age.
   b. The most common pattern of progression is insidious onset.
   c. Schizophrenia in females starts earlier than in males.
   d. Nonpsychotic disturbance can precede psychotic symptoms.
   e. Schizophrenia is rare in childhood when compared with adolescence.

5. Which of the following is *least* helpful in differentiating schizophrenia from pervasive developmental disorder?

   a. Social functioning
   b. Family history of schizophrenia
   c. Hallucinations
   d. Age of onset
   e. Delusions

6. Developmental differences in the DSM-IV-TR criteria for depressive mood disorders in children as compared with adults include all of the following *except:*

   a. Duration of symptoms can be shorter in children for dysthymic disorder.
   b. Diminished ability to concentrate is often due to the presence of delusions.
   c. Depressed mood can include irritable mood.
   d. Major depressive episodes more commonly occur with other comorbid mental disorders.
   e. Failure to gain weight can substitute for change in weight or appetite.

7. Infants who are separated from their primary caregivers and look depressed, cry a lot, react slowly to stimuli, move slowly, and have sleep and appetite disturbances were referred to by Spitz as having:

   a. Endogenous depression
   b. Anticlimactic depression
   c. Atypical depression
   d. Anhedonia
   e. Anaclitic depression

8. All of the following factors may help to predict bipolar disorder in adolescents with major depressive disorder *except:*

   a. Insidious onset of symptoms
   b. Psychomotor retardation
   c. Psychotic features
   d. Psychopharmacologically precipitated mania
   e. Family history of bipolar disorder

9. Medical conditions mimicking depression include all of the following *except:*

   a. Influenza
   b. Asthma
   c. Diabetes
   d. Mononucleosis
   e. Medication side effects

10. Based on recent imaging studies, all of the following statements regarding brain morphology in youth with schizophrenia are correct *except:*

   a. They have decreased total cerebral volume and increased ventricular volume.
   b. They have reduced area of thalamus and cerebellar volume.
   c. They have increased size of corpus callosum.
   d. They have increased size of prefrontal lobe.
   e. They have enlarged lateral temporal lobe.

11. All of the following cytogenetic abnormalities have been reported in patients with childhood onset of schizophrenia *except:*

    a. Turner syndrome
    b. Velocardiofacial syndrome (22q11 deletion)
    c. CGG repeat in FMR1 gene
    d. Translocation of chromosomes 1 and 7
    e. D4 receptor polymorphism

12. All of the following statements are correct regarding the course, prognosis, and outcome of mood disorders in youth *except:*

    a. Both major depressive disorder and bipolar disorder in adolescents increase the risk for suicide.
    b. Youth with early onset depressive disorders have a poorer prognosis and stronger genetic loading.
    c. The age of onset of major depressive disorder has increased over the last 25 years.
    d. Youth with dysthymic disorder have longer episodes and a higher risk for subsequent major depressive episodes.
    e. Depressed youths have increased risk of recurrent mood disorders and other comorbid conditions.

13. All of the statements regarding hallucinations in children are correct *except:*

    a. They are pathognomonic for psychosis.
    b. Auditory hallucinations are the most common ones, followed by visual hallucinations.
    c. Auditory hallucinations in children present similarly to hallucinations in adults.
    d. Long-term follow-up studies indicate that hallucinations are not necessarily associated with an increased risk for major psychiatric disorders.
    e. Hallucinations rarely occur in children under 6 years of age.

14. All of the statements regarding bipolar disorder in youth are correct *except:*

    a. Initial manic symptoms may be less severe in youth than adults.
    b. Most first episodes are hypomania or mania.
    c. Presentations of mania in youth are often atypical.
    d. Irritability and labile mood are more common than euphoria.
    e. Male gender is associated with a higher prevalence of early onset bipolar disorder.

15. The presentation of schizophrenia in adolescence is similar to that in adulthood, whereas the presentation in childhood is said to be different in all of the following ways *except:*

    a. Gradual onset is more common in childhood onset.
    b. Childhood onset is associated with poor outcome.
    c. Premorbid developmental problems of childhood onset schizophrenia are related to severity of long-term outcome.

    d. A subgroup of children with schizophrenic features is called "multidimensionally impaired."
    e. First psychotic episodes in childhood onset are less specific.

16. All of the following statements regarding the premorbid functioning in children who later develop schizophrenia are correct *except:*

    a. The majority of these children display features of pervasive developmental disorders.
    b. One third to half of these children may experience developmental delays and disturbances in language, motor, and social functioning.
    c. Disturbances in adaptive social behavior and withdrawal are considered risk factors.
    d. Many of these children may experience attention-deficit hyperactivity disorder (ADHD)-like symptoms.
    e. These children experience overall greater premorbid impairment compared to the children with major depression.

17. Acute hallucinations in young children can be the result of all of the following *except:*

    a. Hypnagogic or hypnopompic phenomena
    b. Physical illness with fever
    c. Attention deficits and hyperactivity
    d. Acute phobic reactions
    e. Migraine headaches

18. To distinguish the phenomenon of imaginary companions from hallucinations, all of the following statements are correct *except:*

    a. Children with an imaginary companion usually appear to be normal otherwise without showing signs of a thought disorder.
    b. These children can willingly bring out or dismiss their imaginary companions.
    c. The companions are not threatening, discomforting, or distressing to these children.
    d. Persistent hallucinations (not transient imaginary phenomena) are associated with psychopathologies and are pathognomonic of serious psychotic illnesses.
    e. Companions are not ego-alien to these children, who can talk freely about their "friends."

19. All of the following statements related to the neuropsychological functions of children with schizophrenia are correct *except:*

    a. Rote language skills and simple perceptual functions are impaired.
    b. Performance is impaired on fine motor speed tasks that demand attention or short-term memory.
    c. More perseverative errors are made on Wisconsin Card Sorting Tests.
    d. More errors are made on Rey's Tangled Lines—a guided visual search task.
    e. Deficits in auditory attention, verbal memory, and mental flexibility are found.

20. All of the following symptoms might be considered symptoms of depression in children *except:*

    a. Irritability
    b. Loss of interests
    c. Declining school performance
    d. Somatic complaints
    e. Hypersexuality

21. Compared to adolescents, which of the following conditions is the *least* important to be considered in the differential diagnoses of major depressive disorder in preschoolers?

    a. Neglect and abuse
    b. Failure to thrive
    c. Separation anxiety disorder
    d. Schizophrenia
    e. Adjustment disorder with depressed mood

22. All of the following symptoms help to differentiate manic children from those with ADHD *except:*

    a. Elated mood
    b. Push of speech and distractibility
    c. Psychotic symptoms
    d. Grandiosity
    e. Hypersexuality

23. All of the following findings from genetic studies have been reported in bipolar disorder *except:*

    a. Higher concordance for monozygotic twins
    b. Increased depression in biologic relatives
    c. Greater incidence in adopted-out offspring of bipolar parents
    d. The responsible genes have been identified
    e. Association between early onset and increased risk in offspring

24. Regarding the prognosis or outcome of depressive disorders in children and adolescents, all of the following statements accurately reflect current knowledge *except:*

    a. A follow-up study of prepubertal onset major depression showed a threefold increase in suicide attempts.
    b. A longitudinal study of adolescents with depression and anxiety showed twofold to threefold increased risk of adulthood disorders.
    c. Earlier age of onset implies more frequent future episodes and a higher risk of requiring hospitalization.
    d. A majority (approximately 80%) of children and adolescents with major depression have comorbid conditions.
    e. Children comorbid with conduct disorder have a worse outcome of depression.

25. All of the following statements about the epidemiology of mood disorders in children and adolescents accurately represent the current state of knowledge *except:*

    a. Depressive disorder is almost two to three times as prevalent in adolescence as in childhood.

    b. Prepubertal unipolar depression has the same rate in boys and girls.
    c. Prepubertal bipolar disorder has a higher rate in girls.
    d. In adolescents, the rate of unipolar depression in females is twice that in males.
    e. Approximately 20% of first manic episodes occur before the age of 20.

26. Which of the following premorbid conditions is *least* likely seen in patients with early onset schizophrenia?

    a. Language abnormalities
    b. Disruptive behavior
    c. Motor delays
    d. School performance problems
    e. Shyness

27. All of the following statements regarding genetic factors and risk of developing schizophrenia represent the current state of knowledge *except:*

    a. So far studies have failed to verify the association between apolipoprotein E alleles and human leukocyte antigen with childhood onset schizophrenia.
    b. Genetic studies can usually predict who will develop schizophrenia.
    c. Patients with childhood schizophrenia have increased family history of primary psychotic disorders and some personality disorders.
    d. Parents of children with schizophrenia have higher likelihood of carrying diagnoses of schizophrenia and schizotypal personality disorder.
    e. Environmental triggers may play important roles in developing schizophrenia.

28. All of the following are risk factors in the development of schizophrenia *except:*

    a. Pregnancy and birth complications
    b. Female gender
    c. Increased prenatal viral infections in mothers of schizophrenic patients
    d. Neurological soft signs
    e. Abnormalities in autonomic functioning

29. Which of the following conditions is *least* likely to be seen in children and adolescents with schizophrenia?

    a. Hypertonia and hyperreflexia
    b. Smooth pursuit eye movement abnormalities (such as elevated P50 ratio and anticipatory saccades)
    c. Autonomic nervous system abnormal activities in electroencephalograms (EEG)
    d. Progressive brain structural changes during adolescence
    e. Asymmetry patterns of amygdala and hippocampus

30. All of the following statements regarding the prognosis and outcome of early onset schizophrenia are correct *except:*

    a. Earlier onset is associated with better prognosis.
    b. Acute onset is associated with better prognosis.

c. Affective symptoms are associated with better prognosis.

d. Premorbid personality disorders and poor adjustments are associated with poor prognosis.

e. Negative symptoms are less responsive to pharmacological interventions than positive symptoms.

31. All of the following are age-specific clinical characteristics of mania in children compared to adolescents and adults *except:*

a. More emotional lability and irritability

b. More mixed features

c. More rapid cycling

d. More euphoria and elation

e. More comorbid externalizing disorders

32. All of the following statements regarding dysthymic disorder in children and adolescents are correct *except:*

a. Duration of mood symptoms must last a year or longer.

b. Irritable mood can be diagnostic as well as depressed mood.

c. Patients with this diagnosis should not be symptom-free for more than 2 months.

d. The diagnosis cannot be given to patients who had a major depressive episode during the first 2 years of the disturbance.

e. Double depression refers to the occurrence of a subsequent major depressive episode on top of dysthymic disorder.

33. Secondary dysthymia refers to the condition when dysthymia is comorbid with any of the following disorders *except:*

a. Bulimia nervosa

b. Rheumatoid arthritis

c. Somatization disorder

d. Anxiety disorder

e. Psychoactive substance dependence

34. Compared to older adolescents, younger children with major depression may be more likely to experience which of the following symptoms?

a. Depressed mood

b. Lack of concentration

c. Insomnia

d. Somatic complaints

e. More lethal suicide attempts

35. Which of the following medical conditions is *least* likely to mimic mania in children and adolescents?

a. AIDS

b. Seizures

c. Hypothyroidism

d. Multiple sclerosis

e. Wilson's disease

ANSWERS AND EXPLANATIONS

1. (c) According to the DSM-IV-TR, there are hallucinations, delusions, and thought disturbances during the active phase. The duration of illness must be at least 6 months, which may include prodromal or residual symptoms. However, while functioning below the highest level previously achieved is a criterion for adults, in children or adolescents, "failure to achieve the expected level of interpersonal, academic, or occupational achievement" is a diagnostic criterion. *(Ref. 1, pp. 381; Ref. 3, p. 745; Ref. 4, pp. 312–313)*

2. (d) According to adult literature, the average age of onset of schizophrenia is approximately 5 years earlier in males than in females, in the early to mid-20s for males and in the late 20s for females. Overall, the onset of schizophrenia usually occurs between the late teens and the mid-30s. In childhood schizophrenia, boys showed earlier signs of abnormal development and more insidious onset than girls. However, studies did not confirm the gender differences in the onset of schizophrenia among prepubertal patients. *(Ref. 1, pp. 384; Ref. 4, pp. 307–308)*

3. (c) Children with early onset schizophrenia may experience significant developmental deficits in language and motor functioning, with impairment of social functioning. A recent study showed the first signs of dysfunction in the premorbid period are disturbances in adaptive functioning and a tendency for withdrawal. The most common reported positive symptoms are hallucinations. Affective disturbance is reportedly common as well, whereas catatonic symptoms are less frequent. Most children with schizophrenia were found to perform in the low average to average range on the measures of intelligence, with mean IQ between 82 and 94. *(Ref. 1, pp. 386–387; Ref. 3, p. 748)*

4. (c) Studies show childhood schizophrenia is rarely diagnosed before 5 years of age. Among three patterns of onset, the insidious onset pattern is the most common. A study showed nonpsychotic disturbance occurred earlier (4.6 years of age), followed by psychotic symptoms (6.9 years of age), and followed by a full diagnosis of schizophrenia at age 9.5 years. In childhood schizophrenia, early studies showed that boys had earlier signs of abnormal development and more insidious onset than girls. However, a recent study did not confirm the gender differences in the onset of schizophrenia among prepubertal patients. The incidence of schizophrenia increases with age and onset is more likely in the late teens and early adulthood. *(Ref. 1, p. 384; Ref. 3, p. 748; Ref. 4, pp. 307–308)*

5. (a) Social functioning can be impaired in both disorders and is not particularly useful in the differential diagnoses. IQ can help to distinguish autism and childhood onset schizophrenia because many schizophrenic children have low average IQ, but the majority of children with autism are mentally retarded. However, full-scale IQ does not differ between children with childhood schizophrenia and those with high functioning autism. Children with positive family history of schizophrenia may have a higher risk of having schizophrenia, not autism. Unlike schizophrenia, pervasive developmental disorder and autism usually do not have associated hallucinations and delusions. Autism is usually recognized by 3 years of age, while schizophrenia is rarely seen before age 5. *(Ref. 1, pp. 390–391; Ref. 2, p. 126; Ref. 3, pp. 746, 751)*

6. (b) Developmental differences include the following: Only a 1-year duration of dysthymia (also true for cyclothymic disorder) is necessary as compared with 2 years for adults, an irritable or cranky mood can substitute for the depressed mood necessary in adults, and failure to make the expected weight gain can be used for the change in weight or appetite necessary in adults. In children and adolescents, major depressive episodes occur more frequently with other mental disorders. *(Ref. 3, p. 768; Ref. 4, pp. 349–354, 377, 400)*

7. (e) In institutionalized infants and toddlers, this clinical picture has been called anaclitic depression. Once acknowledged, it has led to fewer children being placed in institutions and an effort to find stable caretaking arrangements for children without a psychological parent. *(Ref. 3, p. 769)*

8. (a) A rapid (not insidious) onset of symptoms is more predictive of later manic episodes, among other factors listed. *(Ref. 2, p. 131; Ref. 3, p. 784)*

9. (b) Asthma does not commonly mimic depression. The other conditions listed, as well as thyroid disorders, can present in young people as depression and need to be ruled out in a young person with depressive symptoms. *(Ref. 3, p. 773)*

10. (d) Abnormalities have been found in the structure and function of brains of adults with schizophrenia. Efforts have been made by researchers at NIMH to examine brain morphology of children with schizophrenia. Although replication is needed, some preliminary results indicate several significant differences between children with schizophrenia and control subjects. All of the listed structural differences were found in the NIMH sample except for the size/volume of prefrontal lobes. *(Ref. 3, p. 749)*

11. (c) The etiology of schizophrenia is still controversial and multifactorial, with genetic, neurobiological, environmental, and psychosocial influences. Based on some recent genetic studies, a number of cytogenetic abnormalities were identified in patients with childhood onset schizophrenia. An additional abnormality is the CAG repeat encoded polyglutamine gene. On the other hand, an FMR1 gene mutation with an abnormally high number of CGG repeats is identified in fragile X syndrome and can present with mental retardation, developmental difficulties, ADHD-like symptoms, and autistic features. *(Ref. 1, pp. 235, 393–394)*

12. (c) Based on longitudinal epidemiological studies, the age of onset of major depression has decreased (not increased) over the last 25 years, and early onset predicts overall poorer prognosis and higher genetic predisposition. The average length of a major depressive episode is 9 months and it takes even longer to recover from a dysthymic episode. Dysthymic disorder in youth also predicts an increased risk of having subsequent major depressive episodes and comorbid mental illness. Major mood disorders have significant negative impact on many aspects of youth, causing significant impairments, such as school failure, school dropout, poor interpersonal relationships, decreased global functioning, risk of subsequent alcohol abuse, illicit drug abuse, and suicide, etc. (Ref. 1, pp. 468–469; Ref. 2, pp. 130–131)

13. (a) Hallucinations in younger children (especially under age 6) are rare and not pathognomonic for psychosis. They can occur not only in children with bipolar disorder, depression, personality disorders, and primary psychotic disorders, but also in normal children under stress and in response to transient situations. Children experience a similar spectrum of different types of hallucinations as adults; auditory hallucinations are the most common, followed by visual hallucinations. One long-term follow-up study found continued hallucinations were not associated with an increased risk for later psychopathologies, whereas another indicated that 80% of the subjects with continued hallucinations required further psychiatric care. (Ref. 3, p. 362)

14. (b) For many reasons, it is more difficult and challenging to diagnose bipolar disorders in children and adolescents. Manic symptoms may present with less severe symptomatology and gradually build up over time; this can be misleading and cause underdiagnosing of bipolar disorder. Most adolescents who eventually are diagnosed with bipolar disorder present with depressive episodes or undetermined episodes as their first episodes and less frequently with manic or hypomanic episodes. Patients often initially demonstrate atypical presentations, such as behavioral problems that can mask bipolar disorder. Instead of euphoria, irritability and labile mood states are more common in children and adolescents. Patients with early onset bipolar disorders may experience higher rates of psychotic symptoms, and more male patients are in this group. Early onset is associated with higher incidences of behavior disorders in childhood and substance use disorders at onset, and poor school performance. (Ref. 1, pp. 443–444)

15. (c) Childhood onset schizophrenia is characterized by insidious onset and chronic course with poorer outcome. Some outcome studies have shown that female patients with adolescent onset have better outcome than males. Premorbid functioning and severity of symptoms (both negative and positive) during the acute episodes predicted outcome, whereas studies failed to link severity of outcome with the presence of premorbid developmental problems or premorbid nonpsychotic disturbances. Childhood onset is also associated with less specific initial psychotic episodes presenting with more social withdrawal and antisocial behavior. The disorder termed "multidimensionally impaired" was proposed by McKenna et al. to describe children who present with ADHD-like and psychotic symptoms, but do not meet criteria for schizophrenia. (Ref. 1, pp. 388–391; Ref. 2, pp. 125–126)

16. (a) Premorbid impairments in language, motor, and social functioning have been identified in the developmental histories of children who later developed schizophrenia. Only a subgroup (not a majority) of these children displays autistic-like (pervasive developmental disorder [PDD]) symptoms, such as hand flapping, echolalia, and lack of social responsiveness. Children with premorbid disturbances in adaptive social behavior and tendency for withdrawal are considered to have a higher vulnerability. Depressive symptoms, conduct disturbance, attention deficits and hyperactivity—even ADHD and attention-deficit disorder (ADD) diagnoses—can precede schizophrenia diagnosis in some of these children. Children with early onset schizophrenia have poorer premorbid adjustments and functioning compared to children with major depression. (Ref. 3, p. 748)

17. (c) Illusions and hallucinations can occur normally while falling asleep (hypnagogic) or awakening (hypnopompic). In addition, children can experience hallucinations as a normal reaction to acute phobia and some medical illnesses. ADHD can present as premorbid inattention and hyperactive symptoms or as a diagnosis that precedes the appearance of psychotic symptoms. However, acute hallucinations are not usually the result of attention deficits and hyperactivity. Some other conditions or disorders that need to be considered as differential diagnoses are mood disorders, organic syndromes (often including seizure disorders, central-nervous-system lesions, delirium, metabolic and endocrine disorders, neurodegenerative disorders, developmental disorders, toxic encephalopathies, infectious diseases, and autoimmune disorders), substance abuse, personality disorders, multidimensional impairment, and anxiety disorders. Schizophrenia is a frequent initial misdiagnosis in children and adolescents with bipolar disorder. The combination of disorganized speech and behavior disorder can be confused with schizophrenia in young people. (Ref. 1, pp. 390–393; Ref. 2, p. 127; Ref. 3, p. 880)

18. (d) Persistent hallucinations are frequently associated with serious primary psychotic disorders or psychiatric disorders with psychotic features. However, the hallucinations are not pathognomonic of those disorders, and other conditions need to be considered as differential diagnoses, such as drug intoxication, seizure disorder, metabolic disorders, infections, immaturity, stress, and anxiety. (Please also see question 17.) In normal young children, an imaginary companion phenomenon is not uncommon. (Ref. 3, p. 536)

19. (a) Deficits in attention and processing information have been identified in numerous neuropsychological studies. In addition to the deficits in some areas of spatial organization, except for answer a, all of the listed statements are correct regarding the neuropsychological deficit findings in children with schizophrenia, compared to normal controls. In contrast, the rote language skills and simple perceptual functions are not impaired. (Ref. 3, pp. 749–750)

20. (e) Symptoms that often motivate a parent to seek help for a depressed child include irritability, loss of interest, moodiness, other disruptive behavior, declining school performance, withdrawal from social activities, and somatic complaints (especially headaches and abdominal pain). A correlation between frequency of somatic complaints and severity of depression is reported. Reports also show that depressed young children

might themselves report sadness, suicidal ideations, and sleep disturbances of which their parents may not be aware. Hypersexuality is usually not a sign of depression; rather, it can be considered as one of the cardinal symptoms of mania. *(Ref. 3, pp. 769, 783)*

21. **(d)** It is important to consider age factors in making a more accurate diagnosis of major depressive disorder in children and adolescents. All of the listed conditions should be considered as differential diagnoses in the youngest age group. However, schizophrenia is very rare in younger age groups compared to other listed conditions. Because adolescents have a higher prevalence of schizophrenia, in adolescents who present with major depression, schizophrenia should be considered as one of differential diagnosis in addition to some other conditions, such as alcohol or drug abuse and anxiety disorders. *(Ref. 3, p. 774)*

22. **(b)** It is sometimes difficult to distinguish between ADHD and bipolar disorders. They often have some overlapping symptoms, such as hyperactivity, push of speech, and distractibility. Based on the recent studies by Geller et al., compared to children with ADHD, children with bipolar disorder experienced more of the following cardinal symptoms: elated mood, grandiosity, hypersexuality, decreased need for sleep, flight of ideas, racing thoughts, social intrusiveness, and increased goal-directed activity. Psychotic symptoms are more likely to be seen in bipolar disorder and are not typically seen in ADHD. *(Ref. 3, p. 783)*

23. **(d)** Several twin studies show higher concordance rates in monozygotic twins as compared with the concordance rates in dizygotic twins. In one of the earlier adoption studies, it was found that 31% of those having biologic parents with bipolar disorder were affected, while only 2% of those without genetic loading had the illness. However, two more recent smaller studies showed inconclusive results. That is why there is only limited evidence to support the hypothesis that genetic factors play a more important role in developing bipolar disorders than family and environmental factors. Family studies showed a partial overlapping vulnerability for both bipolar and unipolar depressions and indicated that there is an increased incidence of unipolar depression in biologic relatives of bipolar patients. Compared to adult onset bipolar disorder, childhood onset is associated with greater genetic predisposition and increases the risk of bipolar disorders in the offspring. Despite efforts made, no gene or combination of genes responsible for bipolar disorders has yet been identified. *(Ref. 3, pp. 784–785)*

24. **(e)** A number of recent longitudinal follow-up studies available in the literature indicate overall poorer outcome for early onset major depression than for adult onset illness. They also show increased risks of suicide attempts, and continued depression and anxiety disorders in adulthood. Early onset depression predicts a higher risk of more frequent future episodes and need for hospitalization, and a greater risk of developing or converting to a bipolar disorder. Frequent comorbid conditions further complicate assessment and treatment. Interestingly, a study showed the outcome of depression is not worse in adulthood when comorbid with conduct disorder. Conduct disorder with depression evolved into antisocial personality disorder with the same likelihood as in patients who had conduct disorder without depression. *(Ref. 3, p. 778)*

25. **(c)** All of the statements represent findings from recent studies except for answer **c**. The rate of unipolar depression increases in girls in adolescence to reach the adult ratio of a greater number of females than males. Some reports also suggest higher rates of bipolar disorders in prepubertal boys than girls. *(Ref. 2, pp. 129–130; Ref. 3, pp. 769, 783)*

26. **(e)** The mean age of onset of premorbid symptoms has been reported as 4.6 years. Premorbid symptoms commonly seen in childhood onset schizophrenia include language abnormalities or delays, motor delays, mood lability, social impairment, and a history of autism or pervasive developmental disorder. Shyness does not particularly predict a high likelihood of developing schizophrenia. *(Ref. 1, pp. 381–382; Ref. 3, pp. 747–748)*

27. **(b)** In the past 20 years, family, twin, and adoption studies have strongly suggested that genetic factors contribute to the risk of developing schizophrenia. It is most likely that multiple factors—including environmental influences—interact, each with varying importance in different individuals, to lead eventually to schizophrenic illness. However, genetic studies have not yet developed a way to predict who will develop schizophrenia. *(Ref. 1, p. 394; Ref. 3, p. 749)*

28. **(b)** Perinatal stress and obstetrical complications are more common in the histories of patients with schizophrenia than in those of controls. Either an equal or a predominant male gender ratio was found in clinical studies of schizophrenia in children and adolescent populations. In addition to pubertal development, infectious disease and immunological factors and some other medical conditions and neurological soft signs can all be risk factors for developing schizophrenia. *(Ref. 1, pp. 394–399)*

29. **(a)** Some children with schizophrenia, or at high risk for developing it, have been observed to experience all the listed conditions as well as hypotonia and hyporeflexia. This suggests biological involvement in the pathogenesis and etiology of schizophrenia, especially early onset. Ongoing efforts are still being undertaken to search for specific biological markers of schizophrenia. *(Ref. 3, pp. 748–750)*

30. **(a)** Factors associated with a good prognosis include late onset, acute onset, presence of affective symptoms and schizoaffective presentations, and better premorbid functioning. A number of studies report that early onset of schizophrenia is associated with poorer outcome and prognosis. Similar to the adult population, the positive symptoms experienced by children with schizophrenia are more responsive to psychotropic medications. *(Ref. 3, p. 752)*

31. **(d)** Mania in children presents with more atypical manic symptoms (than adolescents who usually have more similar presentation to adults) with irritability and emotional lability, mixed features, rapid cycling, and higher rates of comorbid conditions, such as externalizing behavioral disorders. Mania in adolescents presents with euphoria, elation, grandiosity, and paranoia. *(Ref. 3, p. 783)*

32. **(d)** In youth, dysthymic disorder can be diagnosed when there is a depressed mood lasting for more than 1 year (2 years in adults) and at least two of the following are present: (1) appetite change; (2) sleep change; (3) decreased energy; (4) low self-esteem; (5) difficulty in making decisions and poor concentration; and (6) feelings of helplessness. The condition is chronic. Irritable mood can replace depressed mood in youth. A major depressive episode in the first year (first 2 years in adults) of the mood disturbance and a history of mania, hypomania, or mixed episode exclude the dysthymic disorder diagnosis. Both adults and youth cannot be symptom free more than 2 months. The subsequent development of a major depressive episode in patients with dysthymic disorder is called double depression. *(Ref. 3, p. 768; Ref. 4, pp. 376–381)*

33. **(a)** Secondary dysthymia is considered when it is coexisting with any of the listed conditions except for bulimia nervosa. Anorexia nervosa can be a coexisting condition as well. *(Ref. 3, p. 768)*

34. **(d)** Depressed mood, lack of concentration, and insomnia can often occur in all age groups. Somatic complaints, separation anxiety, and depressed look tend to decline, whereas anhedonia, psychomotor retardation, lethality of suicide attempts, drug abuse, and delusions tend to increase with increasing age. *(Ref. 1, p. 438)*

35. **(c)** Differential diagnoses of bipolar disorders can be very broad, not only with other psychiatric disorders, but also with numerous medical conditions that can mimic mania in children and adolescents. Except for hypothyroidism, all of the listed conditions, as well as hyperthyroidism, are likely to mimic mania in children and adolescents. *(Ref. 3, p. 785)*

4

DISORDERS OF CONDUCT
AND BEHAVIOR

QUESTIONS

Directions: Select the best response for each of the questions 1–33.

1. Which of the following DSM-IV-TR disorders is *least* likely to be comorbid with attention-deficit hyperactivity disorder (ADHD) based on current research findings?

   a. Oppositional defiant disorder
   b. Bipolar disorders
   c. Specific learning disorders
   d. Pervasive developmental disorder (PDD)
   e. Depressive disorders

2. Which of the following neurotransmitter metabolite abnormalities is *most* frequently found to be associated with violent behaviors?

   a. 5-Hydroxyindoleacetic acid (5-HIAA)
   b. Monoamine oxidase (MAO)
   c. Vanillylmandelic acid (VMA)
   d. Homovanillic acid (HVA)
   e. 3-Methoxy-4-hydroxyphenylglycol (MHPG)

3. Which of the following factors is *least* clearly related to the etiology of violence?

   a. Neurotransmitter function
   b. Intrauterine and perinatal factors
   c. Nurturing environmental factors
   d. Abuse and/or neglect
   e. Genetic abnormalities

4. Based on neuropharmacologic evidence, which of the following neurotransmitter systems is/are *most* likely to be altered in ADHD?

   a. Dopamine and serotonin
   b. Serotonin and norepinephrine
   c. Dopamine and norepinephrine
   d. Only dopamine
   e. Only norepinephrine

5. According to the DSM-IV-TR, ADHD occurs in approximately what percentage of school-age children?

   a. 1 to 2%
   b. 3 to 7%
   c. 7 to 9%
   d. 9 to 11%
   e. 11 to 15%

6. All of the following are considered key elements in the diagnosis of ADHD *except:*

   a. Hyperactivity
   b. Inattention
   c. Learning disability
   d. Impulsivity

   e. Onset before the age of 7 years

7. Which of the following statements about ADHD is *not* characteristic of the disorder according to the DSM-IV-TR?

   a. Individuals with ADHD obtain less schooling than their peers.
   b. Scores on individual IQ tests are comparable to matched children without ADHD.
   c. Minor physical anomalies occur at a higher rate than in the general population.
   d. In many individuals, symptoms attenuate during late adolescence.
   e. There is a higher rate of substance-related disorders and antisocial personality disorder in family members.

8. Which of the following factors is *least* likely to have an influence on the development of ADHD?

   a. Uterine exposure to maternal tobacco and drug use
   b. Malnutrition and neglect
   c. Lead poisoning
   d. Low birth weight
   e. Food additives

9. Approximately what percentage of children with ADHD will continue to show ADHD symptoms or meet criteria for the disorder in adulthood?

   a. 2%
   b. 10%
   c. 18%
   d. 50%
   e. 90%

10. All of the following are characteristics of a child with oppositional defiant disorder (ODD) *except:*

   a. Argumentative and disobedient behavior
   b. Externalization of blame
   c. More prominent problems with familiar people
   d. Frequent comorbidity with conduct disorder
   e. Representation of a long-standing pattern

11. All of the following statements regarding conduct disorder (CD) and related aggressive and violent behaviors are correct *except:*

   a. Prevalence of CD ranges from 1 to 10%.
   b. Prevalence of CD is higher in females.
   c. Violence is associated with extreme poverty.
   d. Violent youth are themselves more likely to be victims of violence.
   e. Aggressive behaviors are associated with large family size and broken homes.

12. All of the following statements regarding the neurological vulnerabilities related to conduct disorder are correct *except:*

    a. Minor head injuries have no relationship with conduct disorder unless they are associated with prolonged unconsciousness.
    b. Certain parts of the brain (such as the temporal lobe and frontal poles) are more vulnerable.
    c. Mild concussions may lead to cognitive impairment.
    d. Any head injury, regardless of which part of the brain is involved, may lead to impairment in judgment and impulse control, and mood instability.
    e. Injuries to the frontal lobe (which is responsible for executive functioning) are associated with poor impulse control and aggressive behaviors.

13. Factors associated with a poor prognosis (such as future violence) in conduct disorder include all of the following *except:*

    a. Fire setting
    b. Violence in childhood
    c. Later age of onset of conduct-disordered behavior
    d. Inattention
    e. Family deviance

14. What percentage of young people with ADHD show a favorable response to stimulant medication?

    a. 40%
    b. 50%
    c. 60%
    d. 75%
    e. 90%

15. Which of the following medications is *least* likely to be considered in the routine treatment of symptoms associated with conduct disorder?

    a. Antidepressants
    b. Valproate
    c. Antipsychotics
    d. Lithium
    e. Benzodiazepines

16. According to available research, which of the following psychosocial interventions has the *least* evidence for the beneficial treatment of conduct disorder as compared with the others listed?

    a. Multisystemic therapy
    b. Family-focused therapy
    c. Individual psychodynamic psychotherapy
    d. Parent management training
    e. Cognitive problem-solving skills training

17. According to the DSM-IV-TR, which of the following is *not* one of the symptoms under criteria A for ADHD?

    a. Often loses things
    b. Often deliberately annoys others
    c. Often interrupts or intrudes on others
    d. Often fails to give close attention to details
    e. Often fidgets

18. Vulnerability factors associated with conduct disorder include all of the following *except:*

    a. Prenatal alcohol and substance abuse by the mother
    b. Temperament
    c. Physical and/or sexual abuse
    d. Family history of antisocial behaviors
    e. Cultural value of dependence

19. All of the following statements regarding laboratory-based research studies on ADHD are correct *except:*

    a. The Continuous Performance Test (CPT) can be used to measure sustained attention.
    b. Measures of attention may not correlate with classroom performance.
    c. The CPT is sensitive to ADHD drug effects.
    d. Measures on the Paired-Associates Learning Task show correlation with blood levels of stimulants.
    e. The CPT is diagnostically specific for the inattention in ADHD.

20. Girls with ADHD demonstrate all of the following differences compared to boys with ADHD *except:*

    a. Lower prevalence rate
    b. Predominantly inattentive type
    c. Higher comorbid rates of anxiety and depression
    d. Higher comorbid rates of disruptive behavior disorders
    e. Greater likelihood of being underdiagnosed

21. All of the following conditions/disorders may contribute to the development of ADHD *except:*

    a. Older mother
    b. Low birth weight
    c. Fetal post maturity
    d. Glucose-6-phosphate dehydrogenase deficiency
    e. Phenylketonuria

22. All of the following statements regarding the evaluation of a child for ADHD are correct *except:*

    a. Symptom ratings should be sought from multiple informants.
    b. Symptoms should be observed and evaluated in different settings.
    c. Neurological soft signs are diagnostic of ADHD.
    d. A recent medical evaluation and examination should be performed.
    e. The child's height and weight should be documented prior to treatment.

23. Which of the following statements regarding the Multimodal Treatment Study of Attention-Deficit Hyperactivity Disorder (MTA study) is *incorrect?*

    a. There were four treatment groups in the study.
    b. It initially included 7- to 9-year-old children with ADHD, combined type.

c. The outcomes of medication treatment and combined treatment were both superior to other treatment groups.

d. Combined treatment had much greater improved outcome than treatment with medication alone.

e. It provided strong evidence to support the efficacy of well-delivered pharmacotherapy for ADHD.

24. Which of the following is *not* a characteristic of ODD?

a. Noncompliance with directions from authority figures

b. Exhibiting more symptoms in front of familiar people

c. Anger being directed mostly toward parents and teachers

d. Physical aggression toward others

e. Defiant behavior taking different forms of expression

25. Which of the following statements regarding intellectual and cognitive vulnerabilities of conduct disorder in children is *not* accurate?

a. Most children with conduct disorder have low to normal or borderline IQ but are not seriously impaired cognitively.

b. The earlier the delinquent behaviors start, the lower is the IQ test performance.

c. Delinquent juveniles have a higher prevalence of learning disabilities.

d. Children with visual–spatial processing deficits have more impaired social skills.

e. Cerebellar dysfunction is highly prevalent in children with conduct disorder.

26. All of the following statements regarding the relationship between abuse and behavioral problems are correct *except:*

a. Early childhood maltreatment is associated with future development of aggressive coping styles.

b. Seriously delinquent and violent juveniles are more likely to be physically abused by their parents.

c. Abuse can be severe, but may not be reported to the authorities.

d. Exposure to domestic violence between parents is also associated with development of aggression and antisocial behavior in their children.

e. Sexual abuse is not associated with aggression.

27. All of the following statements regarding ways of understanding how abuse leads to violence are correct *except:*

a. Children model parental violent behavior.

b. Abuse can result in central nervous system (CNS) damage.

c. Maltreatment can change brain anatomy.

d. Obvious signs of brain dysfunction are found in patients with posttraumatic stress disorder (PTSD) secondary to sexual abuse.

e. A child's rage resulting from parental abuse is displaced from parents onto others, such as the child's teachers and peers.

28. Which of the following is the *least* likely comorbid diagnosis in long-term outcome studies of adolescents with ADHD?

a. Oppositional defiant disorder

b. Major depressive disorder

c. Conduct disorder

d. Schizophrenia

e. Psychoactive substance abuse disorder

29. Which of the following psychotropic medications is *least* likely to be beneficial in the treatment of ADHD?

a. Adderall

b. Strattera

c. Clonidine (Catapres)

d. Lexapro

e. Wellbutrin

30. Psychosocial treatments that have proven efficacious in the management of young people with ADHD include all of the following *except:*

a. Parent training

b. Contingency management

c. Individual psychotherapy

d. Classroom interventions

e. Social skills training

31. Which of the following is the *least* likely long-term educational achievement outcome of adolescents with ADHD?

a. More academic failure

b. Lower education level achieved

c. More learning disabilities

d. Poor performance on certain achievement tests

e. Declining IQ scores

32. All of the following statements regarding stimulant treatment for ADHD are correct *except:*

a. An individual patient will respond equally well to either of the two major categories of stimulants (methylphenidate and dextroamphetamine).

b. In short-term studies, stimulants can help impulse control, attention, and academic and social functioning.

c. A low dose of a stimulant should be initiated and titrated up slowly.

d. Doses in excess of 1.0 mg/kg/day of methylphenidate or 0.5 mg/kg/day of dextroamphetamine require caution.

e. Changing administration timing, dosages, and formulation may help to decrease side effects and wearing-off effects.

33. All of the following features are commonly seen in ODD *except:*

a. Difficult temperament in the preschool years among boys

b. Precocious use of alcohol, tobacco, and drugs

c. Greater prevalence in males during adolescence

d. Greater prevalence in families with multiple caregivers

e. Mothers with depressive disorder more likely to have children with ODD

ANSWERS AND EXPLANATIONS

1. **(d)** Pervasive developmental disorder generally is not found to be comorbid with ADHD. Oppositional defiant disorder, conduct disorder, mood disorders, anxiety disorders, learning disabilities, and Tourette's disorder can all be comorbid with ADHD. Attention-deficit hyperactivity disorder is not diagnosed if inattention and hyperactivity occur exclusively during the course of PDD or a psychotic disorder. *(Ref. 1, pp. 491, 511–512; Ref. 3, pp. 651–655; Ref. 4, pp. 88–91)*

2. **(a)** The neurotransmitter metabolite most frequently associated with violence is 5-HIAA, a serotonin metabolite. Some studies show the association between low cerebrospinal fluid (CSF) levels of 5-HIAA and impulsiveness and aggressiveness. A study of a group of aggressive young boys with ADHD revealed greater serotonergic responsivity. One study also revealed that adolescents with conduct disorder and early onset maladaptive behaviors had higher blood levels of serotonin and the blood levels were associated with ratings of aggressiveness. A recent prospective study in infants also showed modest correlation between initial low CSF 5-HIAA levels (during the first weeks of life) and subsequent aggressive behaviors (at 30 months of age). Both MHPG and VMA are norepinephrine metabolites, and HVA is a dopamine metabolite. *(Ref. 3, pp. 388–389)*

3. **(e)** No genetic abnormalities have been identified that predispose an individual specifically to violent behavior. In the 1960s and 1970s, it was thought that certain chromosomal abnormalities (e.g., XYY and XXY anomalies) were associated with violence, but these conclusions have been questioned. Some twin studies and adoption studies have indicated possible genetic contributions in developing criminal and antisocial behavior, but there is no evidence to support genetic predisposition specific to violence per se; however, the interaction between environment and biological factors such as difficult temperament does correlate with violence. *(Ref. 3, pp. 388–394)*

4. **(c)** There is strong evidence to support the importance of dopaminergic and noradrenergic system involvement in ADHD. Researchers are exploring the relationships between dopamine transporter and dopamine receptor genes (particularly DRD4 and DRD2 genes) and ADHD. One recent positron-emission tomography (PET) study showed a higher accumulation of radioactive fluorodopa tracer in the right midbrain area among some children with ADHD. Another recent study showed that there were higher levels of norepinephrine in the urine of children with ADHD. Stimulant medications such as methylphenidate, amphetamine, and pemoline act primarily on the dopamine system; noradrenergic agents such as clonidine, guanfacine, atomoxetine, and some tricyclic antidepressants demonstrate beneficial effects in the treatment of ADHD, further supporting the important roles of the dopamine and noradrenergic systems in ADHD. *(Ref. 3, pp. 379–380)*

5. **(b)** According to the DSM-IV-TR, the prevalence of ADHD is 3 to 7%. A recent epidemiological review reported a prevalence rate ranging between 1.95 and 14.4%. ADHD is a male-predominant disorder with a male to female ratio of 2–9:1. Rates are also reported to differ across cultures, geographic locations, and age groups, with generally higher rates in school-age children. *(Ref. 1, p. 492; Ref. 4, p. 90)*

6. **(c)** While learning disability is often present with ADHD, its presence is not necessary for the diagnosis. In addition, other common comorbid disorders may include mood disorders, anxiety disorders, and communication disorders. To be diagnosed with ADHD, the patient has to exhibit at least six of the nine symptoms (that cause impairment in two or more settings) under criteria A in the DSM-IV-TR. These symptoms must have been present for at least 6 months, and some of them present before age 7 years. However, the core elements of ADHD continue to be inattention, impulsiveness, and hyperactivity. *(Ref. 1, pp. 488–491; Ref. 4, pp. 83–93)*

7. **(b)** Intellectual development, as measured by individual IQ tests, appears to be somewhat lower in children with this disorder, although there is no evidence that ADHD is related to intellectual subnormality and there is great variability in IQ among children with ADHD. All of the other statements regarding ADHD are characteristics of ADHD according to the DSM-IV-TR. *(Ref. 4, p. 88–90)*

8. **(e)** Food additives have not been shown to be a significant cause of ADHD, but all the other factors listed may contribute to its development. Diet has been proposed as a factor in developing ADHD, but it has not been established. Not eating breakfast has been shown to interfere with children's attention, but it has not been shown to be a significant factor unique to ADHD. *(Ref. 1, pp. 493–494; Ref. 3, pp. 382–383; Ref. 4, p. 88)*

9. **(d)** The number of patients who had ADHD in their youth and persist in showing disabling ADHD symptoms or meeting criteria for the disorder in adulthood varies from 25 to 68%, based on different longitudinal studies. Studies also indicate high rates for developing comorbid conditions, such as personality disorders, mood disorders, and substance use disorder in adulthood, which may also contribute to ongoing impairments. *(Ref. 1, p. 495; Ref. 3, pp. 664–665)*

10. **(d)** When a child's symptoms meet the criteria for conduct disorder, the diagnosis of oppositional defiant disorder is precluded in favor of the conduct disorder diagnosis. Discrete patterns of oppositional behavior may be secondary to other disorders. Oppositional and defiant behavior must be present for at least 6 months to meet the criteria for diagnosis of ODD. *(Ref. 4, pp. 100–102)*

11. **(b)** Conduct disorder (CD), commonly diagnosed in children and adolescents, occurs more in males than in females. There is a wide range of prevalence rates depending on the time and place that the studies were conducted. In general, the prevalence is estimated to be between 1 and 10%, with a higher rate being reported for males. Studies show that extreme poverty,

large family size, broken homes, gang involvement, and socioeconomic deprivation are associated with aggressive and violent behavior. Studies also show that violent youth tend to be victims of violence themselves. Childhood-type conduct disorder usually occurs in males who frequently display aggression, have disturbed peer relationships, and have a poorer prognosis than those with adolescent onset CD. Adolescent onset-type CD has a lower ratio of males to females than does childhood onset type. Males with conduct disorder frequently exhibit stealing, vandalism, and school discipline problems, whereas females are more likely to exhibit lying, truancy, running away, substance use, and prostitution. Females with CD tend to use more nonconfrontational behaviors than males. *(Ref. 2, pp. 43–45; Ref. 3, p. 671; Ref. 4, p. 97)*

12. **(a)** Neurological impairments in children with conduct disorder are usually subtle. In contrast to the former understanding of brain injury, recent studies indicate that minor injuries (even without loss of consciousness) can have a cumulative effect, which can result in cognitive impairments. Even though the frontal and temporal lobes are more vulnerable, brain injuries in any areas of the brain can cause negative consequences, with the frontal lobe being particularly important due to its responsibility for executive functioning. *(Ref. 3, pp. 673–674)*

13. **(c)** Early age of onset of conduct disordered behavior carries a poor prognosis. A history of childhood violence is not necessarily predictive of adult violence in itself. Persistence occurs in up to half of those with conduct disorder at 2-year follow-up and is associated with all of the conditions listed except for answer **c**. Persistence of the symptoms differs between genders. Although data are mixed regarding the gender differences, severity of the conduct disorder predicts persistence of symptoms in both genders. *(Ref. 1, pp. 520–521)*

14. **(d)** Even though currently there are no scientific ways to predict response, the majority (approximately three quarters) of children with ADHD will respond to one of the first-line stimulant medications. The others will likely respond to a higher dose of the same agent or an alternative stimulant. Preschoolers are more prone to side effects and have overall lower response rates. Therefore, slow titration is generally recommended. *(Ref. 2, p. 39; Ref. 3, p. 659)*

15. **(e)** Conduct disorder not only can present with aggression but is also often comorbid with depression, ADHD, and other conditions; may involve concomitant neurologic impairment; and may precede psychosis. Therefore, the medications listed (except for benzodiazepines), as well as stimulants, clonidine, other antipsychotics, and beta-blockers, are commonly considered to target different associated symptoms. Benzodiazepines are rarely indicated for routine treatment of conduct disorder-related symptoms except that they may be used as part of chemical restraint in emergency or crisis situations, especially in an inpatient setting. *(Ref. 1, pp. 519–520; Ref. 3, p. 678)*

16. **(c)** In general, conduct disorder needs a multimodel approach to treatment. No empirical evidence supports the efficacy or effectiveness of individual psychodynamic therapy. Based on research data, problem-solving skills training, family-focused treatments, parent management training, and multisystemic therapy have all been found to be efficacious psychosocial interventions of conduct disorder. *(Ref. 1, pp. 518–519; Ref. 3, pp. 677–678)*

17. **(b)** "Often deliberately annoys others" is one of the symptoms of oppositional defiant disorder. "Often loses things" and "often fails to give close attention to details" are both symptoms for inattention, and "often interrupts or intrudes on others" and "often fidgets" both are symptoms of hyperactivity–impulsivity for the diagnosis of ADHD. *(Ref. 4, pp. 92, 102)*

18. **(e)** Except for the cultural value of dependence, all of the factors listed are found to be associated with conduct disorder. However, the value of being independent rather than being dependent on others is associated with antisocial behavior. In addition, a history of aggression, attention problems, and poor impulse control is associated with conduct disorder, along with central nervous system pathology, head injury, and learning disabilities. *(Ref. 1, pp. 513–517; Ref. 3, pp. 674–675)*

19. **(e)** Some laboratory measures, procedures, and devices have been used in an effort to diagnose ADHD. However, clinicians still need to rely on parents' and teachers' reports, clinical interviews, and direct observations to diagnose ADHD. CPT can be used to measure sustained attention and the results seem to be sensitive to ADHD drug effects and the dosage of the drugs. However, it is not specific for ADHD because attentional dysfunctions measured by CPT can be also seen in other conditions, such as conduct disorder and anxiety disorders. The measures by CPT may not correlate with classroom performance because the test setting can be much less distracting than the classroom. Measures on the Paired-Associates Learning Task also show correlation with blood levels of stimulants. *(Ref. 1, p. 490)*

20. **(d)** Girls constitute 25% of children with ADHD and have overall lower prevalence rates than boys. Girls are more likely to be underdiagnosed and undertreated because they exhibit fewer disruptive problems and experience symptoms of inattention more than hyperactivity, impulsivity, or aggression. However, girls are more likely to have comorbid anxiety and depression. *(Ref. 2, p. 28)*

21. **(a)** There are numerous potential medical contributions to attention-deficit hyperactivity disorder. Maternal age is associated with ADHD, but usually involves a young mother, rather than an older one. All the other answers listed are among those factors or conditions that contribute to ADHD. *(Ref. 2, p. 30)*

22. **(c)** Soft neurologic signs, such as overflow, mirror movements, and problems with laterality and gross and fine motor movements, can be seen in children with ADHD. However, they are nonspecific signs and are not specifically associated with or necessarily present in children with ADHD. It is important to gather information from the school and home, as well as in the office, since parents and teachers have been known to overdiagnose hyperactivity when consulted separately. Attentional problems are likely to appear more pronounced with familiarity and decreased anxiety. A complete medical evaluation and examination may help to reveal some underlying medical

conditions (such as partial deafness and poor vision) that can cause inattentiveness and restlessness. *(Ref. 1, pp. 488–492)*

23. **(d)** Sponsored by the NIMH, the MTA study was a long-term comprehensive treatment study involving a large number of study subjects (579 male and female children, ages 7 to 9), with combined type ADHD, either with or without comorbid disorders such as oppositional defiant disorder (ODD), conduct disorder (CD), and anxiety disorders. All the statements listed are correct except for answer **d**. Even reanalyzed results did not show combined treatment resulted in greater improvement than treatment with medication alone. The combined treatment did show significantly better outcome for the subgroup with comorbid anxiety, ODD, and CD. *(Ref. 1, p. 499; Ref. 3, pp. 661–662)*

24. **(d)** Individuals with oppositional defiant disorder show stubborn, negativistic, and provocative behavior without serious violation of the rights of other people. The defiance of authority and the expression of aggression take different forms, most predominantly by passive means without the more serious physical aggression seen in conduct disorder. Individuals with ODD exhibit more symptoms towards familiar people, and children with ODD are more likely to direct their anger towards their parents and teachers. *(Ref. 2, pp. 55–57)*

25. **(e)** Numerous cognitive vulnerabilities are associated with the development of conduct disorder in children and adolescents, including borderline IQ, learning disabilities, and information-processing deficits. Lower IQ is associated with early presentation of behavioral problems in children with CD. Frontal lobe (not cerebellar) dysfunction is often associated with children with CD leading to impairments of memory, abstract learning, and concentration. *(Ref. 3, p. 674)*

26. **(e)** In addition to intrinsic factors that lead to maladaptation and behavioral problems, especially aggressive behaviors, environmental stressors can also influence youngsters to become more vulnerable to developing an aggressive coping style. Early maltreatment (such as physical abuse, sexual abuse, witnessing domestic violence) is strongly associated with the future development of aggression and antisocial behaviors. Unfortunately, abusive incidents are sometimes kept secret, hidden, and not reported to the authorities. *(Ref. 3, p. 675)*

27. **(d)** Abuse leads to violence through several pathways (for instance, those listed in the questions). Stress from maltreatment changes not only brain physiology, but also anatomy. A recent study found that patients with PTSD secondary to early sexual abuse experience subtle signs of brain dysfunction and abundant neurodevelopmental problems. *(Ref. 3, p. 675)*

28. **(d)** Prospective long-term follow-up studies show overall poor outcome for adolescents who were diagnosed with ADHD as prepubertal children. Compared to the control groups they have more (50% versus 20%) comorbid conditions at follow-ups. In addition to the listed conditions (except for schizophrenia),

they also had higher comorbid rates with anxiety disorders and learning disabilities. *(Ref. 3, p. 663)*

29. **(d)** Stimulants are still the first line of treatment for ADHD. Alternatives may include Strattera, Clonidine, Tenex, and Wellbutrin, among others. However, SSRIs have not been found effective in treating core symptoms of ADHD, although they can be considered in the treatment of comorbid conditions such as depression and anxiety. *(Ref. 1, pp. 495–498; Ref. 3, pp. 659–661)*

30. **(c)** There are no empiric data to support efficacy of individual psychotherapy for ADHD core symptoms. All of the other interventions listed are empirically proven efficacious as ADHD treatment modalities. Psychosocial interventions are important components of comprehensive treatment for ADHD, especially because ADHD is a complex disorder that affects many aspects of patients' and their families' lives. Because psychosocial interventions show weak effects on the core symptoms of ADHD, treatments combined with medication are recommended. Psychosocial interventions can help parents learn to manage patients' behavioral problems, help patients deal with peer relations, and help to decrease family dysfunction. *(Ref. 3, pp. 657–659)*

31. **(e)** Long-term prospective studies have shown overall poor educational outcome for adolescents who were diagnosed with ADHD when they were younger. Studies have concluded that academic difficulties, including poor grades, lower level of education, poor performance on achievement tests for reading and arithmetic, and a high prevalence of learning disabilities, continued from elementary school to high school. No data indicated the decline of IQ in these studies, although children with low IQ (below 80) were excluded from some of the studies. *(Ref. 3, pp. 662–663)*

32. **(a)** Stimulants are still the first line of treatment for ADHD. The most commonly used are methylphenidate agents such as Ritalin, dextroamphetamine agents such as Dexedrine, or mixed-salts agents such as Adderall. Individuals may respond uniquely to different stimulants even though overall response rate is high (75% of children respond to the first medications tried). A trial of an alternative medication may be necessary for those who do not respond to the first stimulant tried. To minimize side effects, a low starting dose and slow titration are recommended. Using higher doses, such as >1.0 mg/kg/day (or 60 mg/day) of methylphenidate or >0.5 mg/kg/day (or 30 mg/day) of dextroamphetamine, requires extra caution. Changing the administration schedules, dosages, and formulations (such as using longer acting formulations) may help to decrease wearing-off and side effects from the stimulants. *(Ref. 3, p. 659)*

33. **(c)** According to the DSM-IV-TR, ODD is more prevalent in males than in females before puberty, but the rates are nearly equal after puberty. All of the other features listed are found in ODD. *(Ref. 4, pp. 100–101)*

5

ANXIETY DISORDERS (INCLUDING SEPARATION ANXIETY, OVERANXIOUS AND AVOIDANT DISORDERS, OBSESSIVE–COMPULSIVE DISORDER, PHOBIA, AND POSTTRAUMATIC STRESS DISORDER)

QUESTIONS

Directions: Select the best response for each of the questions 1–34.

1. Which of the following best describes the DSM-IV-TR characterization of separation anxiety disorder?
   a. Excessive anxiety and apprehensive expectations that make a child anxious and preoccupied.
   b. Markedly disturbed and developmentally inappropriate social relatedness.
   c. Excessive anxiety about being apart from the individuals to whom the child is most attached.
   d. A maladaptive response to an identifiable stressor.
   e. Significant anxiety provoked by social or performance situations.

2. The most common cause of school absenteeism is:
   a. Separation anxiety disorder
   b. Conduct disorder
   c. Substance abuse
   d. School phobia
   e. Mood disorder

3. Besides another anxiety disorder, the most common comorbid diagnosis with anxiety disorders in youth is:
   a. Depressive disorders
   b. Phobic disorder
   c. Panic disorder
   d. Obsessive–compulsive disorder (OCD)
   e. Oppositional defiant disorder

4. The differential diagnosis among separation anxiety disorder, generalized anxiety disorder (GAD), panic disorder, and social phobia is best determined by which one of the following?
   a. Age of onset
   b. Underlying etiology
   c. Severity of the symptoms
   d. Presence of somatic complaints
   e. Focus of the anxiety

5. The key to successful therapy for separation anxiety disorder (SAD) resulting in school refusal is best described by which of the following?
   a. Antidepressant treatment
   b. Behavioral therapy
   c. Prompt return to school
   d. Social skills training
   e. Family therapy

6. The most frequent presenting symptom for young people with OCD is:
   a. Counting

   b. Cleaning
   c. Checking
   d. Ego-dystonic thoughts of violence or sex
   e. Hoarding

7. Which of the following mechanisms represents the most likely description of the etiology of OCD?
   a. Child-rearing practices
   b. Modeling
   c. Possession
   d. Genetic and neurobiological contributions
   e. Parental perfectionism

8. Which of the following neurotransmitters is most implicated in the genesis of OCD?
   a. Epinephrine
   b. Norepinephrine
   c. Dopamine
   d. Acetylcholine
   e. Serotonin

9. According to DMS-IV-TR, which of the following percentage ranges represents the prevalence rate of specific phobia in a community sample?
   a. 0.5 to 2%
   b. 4 to 9%
   c. 12 to 18%
   d. 19 to 24%
   e. 25 to 30%

10. Which one of the following phobias is more common in adolescents than in children?
    a. Stranger phobia
    b. Social phobia
    c. School phobia
    d. Blood phobia
    e. Bodily injury phobia

11. The symptoms of posttraumatic stress disorder (PTSD) in children differ from those seen in adults in all of the following ways *except:*
    a. Fear of separation
    b. Reenactment in actual behavior
    c. Reenactment in symbolic activities
    d. Less denial, repression, and psychic numbing
    e. Nightmares and daydreams

12. Obsessive–compulsive disorder in children is *least* likely to be associated with which of the following disorders?
    a. Trichotillomania
    b. Tourette's disorder

c. Nail biting
d. Sydenham's chorea
e. Mental retardation

13. Which of the following is *least* likely to present in children with SAD?

a. Sleep disturbance
b. Excessive fears
c. School absenteeism
d. Ritualistic behavior
e. Somatic complaints

14. All of the following statements are accurate descriptions of the current knowledge about SAD *except:*

a. The disorder is more frequent in males in community-based studies.
b. Adolescents may deny anxiety about separation.
c. Specific fears or concerns (such as about death and dying) are common.
d. Onset must be before the age of 18.
e. Sons of mothers with panic disorder are more likely to have SAD.

15. Which of the following is *least* likely to be an accurate description of most children with GAD?

a. Excessive worry about future events
b. Pseudomaturity
c. Being pessimistic
d. Avoiding social contact
e. Somatic complaints

16. Which of the following statements describing characteristics of separation anxiety disorder and generalized anxiety disorder is false?

a. Separation anxiety disorder occurs more in younger children.
b. Generalized anxiety disorder occurs more commonly in children from a single-parent home.
c. Parents of children with anxiety disorders are significantly more likely to be depressed or anxious.
d. Parents of children with separation anxiety disorder are significantly more likely to have panic disorder.
e. Females have higher prevalence rates for anxiety disorders than males.

17. All the following statements regarding the etiology of anxiety disorders are correct *except:*

a. Anxious temperament may have a genetic basis.
b. Shy, inhibited temperament is a risk factor for developing anxiety symptoms.
c. Highly reactive temperament is a synergistic risk factor with the shy, inhibited temperament for developing anxiety symptoms.
d. Insecure attachment is a risk factor for developing anxiety disorders.
e. Anxious-resistant attachment is associated with developing anxiety disorders in adolescents.

18. Which one of the following medications has been reported to produce symptoms of both separation anxiety and school phobia?

a. Risperidone
b. Imipramine
c. Fluoxetine
d. Alprazolam
e. Sertraline

19. All of the following statements regarding the long-term prognosis for anxiety disorders in childhood are accurate *except:*

a. The majority of children with GAD or SAD recover.
b. Children with anxiety disorders have higher risk of developing other psychiatric illness over time.
c. Young adults with a history of anxiety disorder comorbid with depression are less likely to be employed.
d. A prospective study shows that separation anxiety disorder in childhood predisposes to developing panic disorder in adulthood.
e. Further studies are needed to address long-term outcome of anxiety disorders.

20. Which of the following physical conditions is *least* likely to mimic anxiety disorders in childhood?

a. Hypoglycemic episodes
b. Hypothyroidism
c. Caffeinism
d. Lupus
e. Pheochromocytoma

21. All of the following statements regarding diagnosis of OCD in children are accurate *except:*

a. Patients may experience deterioration of school performance.
b. Patients can be very secretive about their symptoms.
c. Patients usually recognize that obsessions or compulsions are excessive or unreasonable.
d. Symptoms from children with OCD may not be ego-dystonic.
e. Prepubertal onset OCD may be associated with Group A beta-hemolytic streptococcal infection.

22. All of the following statements regarding the epidemiology of OCD in children and adolescents are accurate *except:*

a. Based on community studies, lifetime prevalence rate of OCD in children and adolescents is between 1 and 2.3%.
b. Compulsions are more dominant symptoms in younger children.
c. It has an earlier age of onset in girls.
d. Prevalence rates are more equal in adolescents and adults.
e. Children with early onset OCD are more likely to have a family history of OCD or tic disorder.

23. Which of the following areas of the brain has been found to be dysfunctional in OCD patients?

a. Cerebellum
b. Hippocampus

c. Basal ganglia

d. Parietal lobe

e. Amygdala

24. All of the following statements regarding the long-term prognosis of OCD are correct based on follow-up studies *except:*

    a. Over half of young people with OCD continue to have OCD symptoms into adulthood.

    b. Some young people with OCD go on to develop obsessive–compulsive personality disorder (OCPD).

    c. About one-quarter of young people with OCD are diagnosis free as adults.

    d. The most frequent additional diagnosis at follow-up is depression or anxiety.

    e. Positive response to clomipramine therapy predicts outcome.

25. All of the following are characteristics of young people with specific phobias *except:*

    a. They have persistent fears of a circumscribed stimulus.

    b. They fear having a panic attack.

    c. They have significant anxiety when faced with the feared object or situation.

    d. Fear can interfere with a child's normal routine or cause marked distress.

    e. Young children may not recognize their fear as excessive.

26. The more common fears in prepubertal children include all of the following *except:*

    a. The dark

    b. Animals

    c. Thunder and lightning

    d. Tests in school

    e. Bodily injury

27. All of the following statements regarding the prognosis for phobias are accurate *except:*

    a. Selective mutism usually does not resolve without treatment.

    b. Social phobia has a chronic, unremitting course.

    c. Most simple phobias improve.

    d. Phobic disorders are commonly found in association with other anxiety disorders.

    e. Panic disorder is often chronic or recurrent.

28. All of the following statements regarding panic disorder in children and adolescents are accurate reflections of the current knowledge *except:*

    a. Young children can commonly experience panic symptoms that are associated with another anxiety disorder.

    b. The modal age of onset for classic panic disorder is in latency.

    c. Adolescents with panic disorder commonly report panic symptoms including trembling, dizziness, pounding heart, and shortness of breath.

    d. Panic disorder in children and adolescents is highly associated with separation anxiety disorder.

    e. Adolescents with panic disorder report more somatic symptoms than cognitive ones.

29. All of the following are necessary to establish the diagnosis of PTSD according to the DSM-IV-TR *except:*

    a. Exposure to a traumatic stressor

    b. Reexperiencing

    c. Avoidance, numbing, or lack of responsiveness

    d. Duration of symptoms for more than 6 months

    e. Persistent increased arousal

30. Symptoms commonly seen in young children with PTSD include all of the following *except:*

    a. Difficulty modulating aggression

    b. Withdrawal from new experiences

    c. Flashbacks

    d. Perceptual distortions

    e. Traumatic play

31. Posttraumatic stress disorder may co-occur with all of the following comorbid disorders *except:*

    a. Substance abuse disorders

    b. Conduct disorder

    c. Depression

    d. OCD

    e. Acute stress disorder

32. Chronic or repetitive trauma is most associated with all of the following *except:*

    a. Excessive emotional responsiveness

    b. Interpersonal avoidant behavior

    c. Dissociative responses

    d. Self-mutilation

    e. Heightened arousal

33. All of the following statements regarding factors that affect children's responses to trauma are correct *except:*

    a. Very young children with limited cognitive capacity can respond to trauma.

    b. Higher intelligence is a protective factor.

    c. Preexisting anxiety and depression affect negatively on trauma response in children.

    d. Prior trauma increases the likelihood of children expressing more fear.

    e. Exposed to similar trauma, children's reactions may be different from their parents'.

34. Which of the following disorders is more commonly found to be comorbid with separation anxiety disorder?

    a. Pervasive development disorder, not otherwise specified

    b. Panic disorder with agoraphobia

    c. Schizophrenia

    d. Major depressive disorder

    e. Autism

ANSWERS AND EXPLANATIONS

1. **(c)** Answer **(a)** characterizes generalized anxiety disorder; **(b)** characterizes reactive attachment disorder or pervasive developmental disorder; **(d)** characterizes adjustment disorder; and **(e)** characterizes social phobia. (*Ref. 1, pp. 558–559, 590, 769; Ref. 4, pp. 121–125, 456, 476*)

2. **(b)** Not all children with school absenteeism have separation anxiety, nor do all children with separation anxiety have school absenteeism. Truancy associated with conduct disorder is the most common cause of school absenteeism. Other causes of school absenteeism include those disorders listed, along with mood disorder, panic disorder, OCD, psychotic disorders, realistic fears of harm or humiliation, and parental permission. (*Ref. 2, pp. 65, 68*)

3. **(a)** Anxiety disorders in youth infrequently occur alone with high rates of comorbid conditions. In addition to another anxiety disorder, youth with anxiety disorders are most likely to have a comorbid depressive disorder. A recent study showed 79% of children with an anxiety disorder have at least one of the other conditions. Social phobia, simple phobia, and other externalizing disorders, such as ADHD, are common comorbid diagnoses. (*Ref. 1, p. 560; Ref. 3, p. 823*)

4. **(e)** In generalized anxiety disorder, the anxiety is focused on performance and nonspecific worries about the future. In separation anxiety, the anxiety is focused on separation from attachment figures. In social phobia, the anxiety is focused on being in social situations. In panic attacks, the anxiety is focused on the fear of having another panic attack. (*Ref. 1, pp. 560–561; Ref. 4, pp. 430–475*)

5. **(c)** While all of the treatments listed may be of benefit in the treatment of separation anxiety disorder, a prompt return to school is the most important. The longer the child is out of school, the greater is the likelihood of treatment resistance and chronicity. (*Ref. 2, pp. 68–70*)

6. **(b)** All of the symptoms listed are common in children with OCD, but cleaning (hand washing, showering, bathing, and tooth brushing) is most common, occurring in approximately 85% of these children. Repeating rituals and checking behaviors are also common. (*Ref. 1, pp. 576–577*)

7. **(d)** There is little evidence that OCD is caused by overly strict parenting (toilet training and perfectionism) or by modeling or possession. Genetic mechanisms and neurobiological contributions interacting with environmental factors are the most likely causes of OCD. (*Ref. 1, pp. 579–580; Ref. 2, p. 150; Ref. 3, pp. 836–840*)

8. **(e)** Serotonin reuptake blockers such as clomipramine, fluoxetine, and fluvoxamine are effective in the treatment of OCD, giving strong support to the role of serotonin in the genesis of OCD, although other neurotransmitters may also play a role. (*Ref. 1, p. 579; Ref. 2, p. 150; Ref. 3, p. 838*)

9. **(b)** Fears and anxiety commonly present in children and adolescents with some developmental differences. They present with different patterns in different age groups. The diagnosis of anxiety disorder frequently depends on whether fears and anxiety cause sufficient impairment or distress. Prevalence of specific phobia varies, ranging from 4 to 8.8% in a community sample based on DMS-IV-TR, with a lifetime prevalence range between 7.2 and 11.3%. (*Ref. 2, p. 136; Ref. 3, p. 822; Ref. 4, p. 447*)

10. **(b)** Social phobia seems to begin between 15 and 20 years of age, although there are few studies of children with social phobia. The other disorders listed are more common in children than in adolescents. (*Ref. 2, pp. 137–138*)

11. **(e)** Nightmares and daydreams occur both in children and in adults with PTSD, although the content may be less recognizable with youth. Children are more likely to fear being separated from caretakers, to exhibit traumatic play, and to have less use of defenses, such as denial, repression, and psychic numbing. Instead of experiencing flashback, they may reenact in actual behavior from which they are unable to distinguish with the real events. Regression is more common, as is somatization. (*Ref. 1, pp. 614–616; Ref. 2, pp. 144–145; Ref. 4, p. 466*)

12. **(e)** No data indicate mental retardation is associated with OCD. Obsessive–compulsive disorder is found to be associated with eating–disorders, paraphilias, kleptomania, compulsive gambling, trichotillomania (compulsive hair pulling), and onychophagia (pathological nail biting). It is also found to be associated with basal ganglia disorders, such as Tourette's disorder, Sydenham's chorea, and Huntington's chorea. In addition, OCD is found to be associated with major depression, anxiety disorder, alcohol/substance abuse, conduct/dispositional disorder, and ADHD. (*Ref. 1, pp. 577–578; Ref. 2, p. 150; Ref. 4, pp. 458–459*)

13. **(d)** Ritualistic behavior often presents in youth with OCD and is not commonly seen in SAD. Worries focus on the fear that harm might come to the attachment figure, which often manifest in fears of being apart, such as when going to school or to bed. Complaints or experiencing somatic symptoms (e.g., stomachaches, headaches) are common. (*Ref. 1, p. 558; Ref. 2, pp. 63–65; Ref. 3, p. 824*)

14. **(a)** Adolescents with the disorder, especially males, may deny anxiety about separation, but will have limited independent activity. In clinic samples males and females have equal prevalence, whereas epidemiological data showed higher prevalence in females. Children with separation anxiety disorder tend to come from families where mothers have panic disorder. Differentiation of SAD from certain cultural values (such as independence) emphasized by some families is important. (*Ref. 4, pp. 121–123*)

15. **(d)** While they worry about social acceptability and are pessimistic, children with GAD do enjoy social contact. They may appear "overly mature" since they are perfectionistic and

compliant. They may also show habit disturbances, such as nail biting and hair pulling, and have somatic complaints. *(Ref. 2, p. 140; Ref. 4, pp. 472–474)*

16. **(b)** Generalized anxiety disorder occurs more in adolescents and in those who come from upper socioeconomic backgrounds as compared with separation anxiety disorder, which occurs more in single-parent homes. Separation anxiety occurs more in younger children. Prevalence rates of both SAD and GAD are higher in females. Parents of children with separation anxiety disorder are more likely to have panic disorder and major depression themselves. Studies also show children of parents who have depression and anxiety are more likely to develop an anxiety disorder, with parental anxiety being a strong risk factor. *(Ref. 1, pp. 561–563; Ref. 2, p. 140)*

17. **(c)** Several important domains (such as genetic/temperament, attachment, parental anxiety, parenting style, and life experience) need to be considered as potential interacting factors contributing to the etiology of anxiety disorders. Studies show that shy, inhibited temperament is a risk factor for developing anxiety symptoms with no additional risk if combined with highly reactive temperament. While insecure attachment can be a contributing factor, anxious-resistant attachment is also associated with developing anxiety disorders in adolescents. In addition, parental anxiety, controlling parenting style, and exposure to negative life events are all risk factors for developing anxiety disorders. *(Ref. 1, pp. 561–564)*

18. **(a)** Neuroleptics such as haloperidol, pimozide, and, most recently, risperidone have been reported to cause school phobias in children, described in the past as neuroleptic separation anxiety disorder. First-line pharmacological treatment of SAD is SSRIs, such as fluoxetine and sertraline. Studies show superiority of combined treatment of cognitive–behavioral therapy (CBT) with imipramine over CBT plus placebo. Although benzodiazepines (such as alprazolam) may be effective when used in children before painful medical procedures, studies did not show the efficacy of using benzodiazepines in treating separation anxiety and school phobia over placebo. *(Ref. 1, pp. 564–567; Ref. 2, p. 70; Ref. 3, p. 829)*

19. **(d)** From the follow-up data available, it is possible to say that there is a greater risk for additional psychiatric disorders in adults who had generalized anxiety disorder during their childhood and the majority of children with anxiety disorders do recover over time. Comorbidity with depression increases risk of negative outcomes, such as being less likely to be employed or in school, higher utilization of mental health services, and more psychological problems. The relationship between childhood SAD and adult panic disorder is controversial; more long-term prospective outcome studies are needed. *(Ref. 1, pp. 568–569)*

20. **(b)** All of the conditions listed (except for hypothyroidism) can mimic anxiety symptoms. In addition, other physical conditions to be considered in the differential diagnosis of anxiety disorders include substance intoxication or withdrawal, asthma, use of stimulants, gastrointestinal problems, seizure disorders, cardiac conditions, hyperparathyroidism, hyperthy-

roidism, vestibular dysfunctions, etc. *(Ref. 2, p. 143; Ref. 3, pp. 827–828)*

21. **(c)** Based on DSM-IV-TR, criterion B of OCD—recognition of symptoms as excessive or unreasonable—does not apply to children. While young children may not recognize that the obsessive and compulsive behavior is excessive or unreasonable, children with OCD may or may not be distressed or egodystonic about their symptoms and are often secretive about them. School performance may gradually decline mostly due to impaired concentration. Group A beta-hemolytic streptococcal infection is linked to early onset OCD. *(Ref. 1, pp. 575–576; Ref. 4, pp. 459–463)*

22. **(c)** The age of onset is younger in boys than in girls and prevalence rates become more equal in adolescents and adults. Early onset is also associated with family history of OCD and tic disorder. Obsessive–compulsive disorder is more common than usually thought, occurring with a lifetime prevalence rate of 1 to 2.3% for children and adolescents in community samples. Obsessions or compulsions are known to occur alone, but younger children usually experience more compulsions than obsessions. *(Ref. 1, pp. 576–577; Ref. 4, p. 460)*

23. **(c)** While the etiology of OCD is unknown, it appears to be the result of a frontal lobe-limbic-basal ganglia dysfunction. Neuroimaging, positron-emission tomography studies, computed tomography scans, and neuropsychological testing have all shown abnormalities in the frontal lobe and the basal ganglia. *(Ref. 1, p. 579; Ref. 3, pp. 837–839)*

24. **(e)** The initial baseline measures and response to clomipramine are not associated with outcome. With limited available long-term outcome data, some follow-up studies show at least half of children continue to have OCD symptoms as adults, and approximately half develop additional disorders (more often depression or anxiety), with about one quarter of patients no longer meeting criteria for OCD. Children with early onset OCD may develop OCPD, although the relationship between OCD and OCPD needs further study. *(Ref. 1, p. 584)*

25. **(b)** The fear of having a panic attack is characteristic of panic disorder, which is not characteristic of specific phobia. All other statements correctly describe the characteristics of specific phobia in young people. *(Ref. 1, pp. 589–590)*

26. **(d)** Fears of loud noises, the dark, animals, imaginary creatures, bodily injury, and separation from caregivers are common in younger children. In older children and adolescents, fears are more focused on health, social, and school problems. Certain fears are not considered phobias unless they cause significant functional impairment. *(Ref. 1, pp. 591–592; Ref. 2, pp. 136–137)*

27. **(a)** Regardless of whether receiving or not receiving treatment, selective mutism symptoms tend to remit, although most of these children eventually develop social phobia. While little is known about how children with phobias do later in life, one study found that 80% were symptom free at 2-year follow-up, but 7% had serious fear reactions. Longitudinal studies in adults show panic disorder and social anxiety disorder have a chronic course. *(Ref. 1, p. 602)*

28. **(b)** Panic disorder (especially panic symptoms that are commonly associated with another anxiety disorder) can start in childhood, with a modal age of onset in midadolescence for a full-blown panic disorder that meets DSM criteria. Numerous studies show association between panic disorder in children and adolescents and separation anxiety disorder. Cognitive symptoms are less commonly reported by adolescents with panic disorder than somatic ones, such as trembling, dizziness, pounding heart, nausea, shortness of breath, and sweating. *(Ref. 1, pp. 593–594; Ref. 3, pp. 827–828)*

29. **(d)** All of the symptoms listed are necessary to establish the diagnosis, except for answer **(d)** Duration of the disturbance should be more than 1 month. The DSM-IV-TR criteria are the same for children and adolescents as they are for adults, but intense fear, helplessness, and horror may be expressed in children by disorganized or agitated behavior. *(Ref. 4, pp. 463–468)*

30. **(c)** Flashbacks are far less common in children than in adults. Children are much more likely to reexperience the event through traumatic (symbolic) play or actual behavior. Perceptual distortions are most frequent in the sense of time and vision, but auditory, olfactory, and touch misperceptions also occur. Children with PTSD may appear aloof and withdrawal and dysregulation of hyperarousal can lead to irritability, anger outbursts, and aggression. *(Ref. 1, pp. 610–616; Ref. 2, pp. 144–145)*

31. **(e)** Posttraumatic stress disorder can underlie presentations of psychosis, oppositional defiant disorder, depression, phobias, substance abuse, conduct disorder, anxiety disorders, somatization disorder, or ADHD. Obsessions and compulsions may occur in an effort to control anxiety after a traumatic stressor. An acute stress disorder is replaced by a diagnosis of PTSD when the duration is more than 1 month. The two diagnoses are exclusive to each other. *(Ref. 1, pp. 619–621; Ref. 4, pp. 467–469)*

32. **(a)** Chronic or repetitive trauma is associated with restricted emotional responsiveness. Recurrent or repeated trauma may be an antecedent to borderline personality disorder and all the other symptoms listed. Other possible behaviors include suicide attempts, antisocial behavior, and sexual promiscuity, especially when the traumatic event involved sexual abuse. *(Ref. 3, pp. 915–917; Ref. 4, pp. 464–465)*

33. **(d)** While studies show variable results regarding the gender differences on symptomatic response to trauma, the age factor is also complex. Studies show even younger children with limited cognitive capacity are able to respond to trauma despite less understanding of the danger associated with a stressor. High intelligence is protective, whereas history of academic problems is a risk factor. While preexisting depression and anxiety are associated with heightened reactions to trauma, prior trauma may diminish children's fear reactions and behavioral reenactments. *(Ref. 3, p. 916)*

34. **(d)** Dysthymic disorder and major depressive disorder are frequent comorbid diagnoses with separation anxiety disorder. According to the DSM-IV-TR, separation anxiety disorder is not diagnosed if the symptoms occur during the course of a pervasive development disorder, schizophrenia, or other psychotic disorder or are not better accounted for by panic disorder with agoraphobia, although it may precede them in adolescents and adults. The relationship between SAD and panic disorder is not clear; some researchers think they may represent a common underlying disorder with different clinical presentations. However, based on DSM-IV-TR, they are diagnostically exclusive. *(Ref. 1, p. 593; Ref. 4, pp. 122–125, 449–450)*

6

EATING AND NUTRITIONAL DISORDERS

QUESTIONS

Directions: Select the best response for each of the questions 1–33.

1. Patients with anorexia nervosa (AN) exhibit a number of neuroendocrine abnormalities. All of the following hormonal abnormalities have been found in emaciated patients with anorexia nervosa *except:*
   a. Increased corticotropin-releasing hormone (CTRH)
   b. Increased triiodothyronine (T3)
   c. Blunted diurnal cortisol levels
   d. Decreased estrogens
   e. Decreased luteinizing hormone-releasing hormone (LHRH)

2. All of the following characteristics regarding "Feeding Disorder of Infancy or Early Childhood" are correct *except:*
   a. Onset before 6 years of age
   b. Frequent association with medical disorders such as esophageal reflux
   c. Significant failure to gain or maintain weight
   d. Difficulties with attachment
   e. Difficulties with homeostasis

3. Infantile anorexia nervosa is characterized by all of the following *except:*
   a. Food refusal or selectivity
   b. Onset between 6 months and 3 years of age
   c. Overly indulgent parents
   d. Confusion of somatic and psychological states
   e. Struggles for control between the infant and the caregiver

4. What percentage of healthy young children is reported to have significant feeding problems?
   a. 5%
   b. 15%
   c. 25%
   d. 35%
   e. 50%

5. What approximate percentage of patients with anorexia nervosa develops bulimia nervosa (BN) during the course of the disorder?
   a. 5%
   b. 10%
   c. 25%
   d. 40%
   e. 60%

6. Which of the following physical symptoms is *least* commonly seen in patients with anorexia nervosa, restricting type?
   a. Salivary-gland enlargement
   b. Lanugo hair
   c. Hypercarotenemia
   d. Hypercholesterolemia
   e. Bradycardia

7. Which of the following is the most common psychiatric disorder accompanying anorexia nervosa?
   a. Anxiety disorder
   b. Depressive disorder
   c. Obsessive–compulsive disorder
   d. Personality disorder
   e. Psychotic disorder

8. The first step in treating low-weight adolescent patients with anorexia nervosa is:
   a. Establishment of rapport
   b. Stabilization of the family
   c. Nutritional restoration
   d. Inpatient psychiatric hospitalization
   e. Inpatient pediatric hospitalization

9. The ultimate target weight for an anorexic patient should be based on which of the following?
   a. Enough body weight for the restoration of menses
   b. The ideal body weight as based on published, standardized tables
   c. The patient's ideal weight for herself
   d. The family's ideal weight for the patient
   e. The weight of the patient prior to the onset of the anorexia nervosa

10. The peak time for the onset of BN is:
    a. Preadolescence
    b. Early adolescence
    c. Middle adolescence
    d. Late adolescence
    e. Middle adulthood

11. Many physical disorders have clinical symptoms in common with anorexia nervosa. Which of the following is *least* likely to be considered in the differential diagnosis?
    a. Crohn's disease
    b. Diabetes mellitus
    c. Inflammatory bowel disease
    d. Thyroid disease
    e. Prader–Willi syndrome

12. The prevalence rate of obesity in preschool children is:
    a. 5 to 10%
    b. 15 to 20%
    c. 25 to 30%

d. 35 to 40%

e. 40 to 45%

13. Obesity in females is *more* likely in which social class?

    a. Lower social class
    b. Lower middle social class
    c. Middle social class
    d. Upper middle social class
    e. Upper social class

14. Which of the following medical complications of childhood obesity is potentially the most serious and in need of the most vigorous treatment?

    a. Diabetes mellitus
    b. Hypertension
    c. Slipped femoral epiphysis
    d. Cardiomegaly
    e. Pickwickian syndrome

15. All of the following statements regarding the course and outcome of AN and BN are accurate reflections of the current research literature *except:*

    a. Studies show that AN can be chronic with high relapse rate.
    b. The mortality rate of young women with AN is 12 times as high as that of the general population.
    c. Comorbid with cluster B personality disorders, BN has a poorer prognosis.
    d. Early age of onset is associated with a worse prognosis for BN.
    e. Low serum albumin and low body weight predict a higher mortality rate for AN.

16. All of the following statements regarding pharmacological treatments for anorexia nervosa in adolescents are correct based on current research *except:*

    a. Fluoxetine improves treatment outcome for anorexic inpatients.
    b. SSRIs may help weight-recovered anorexic patients to maintain their weight.
    c. Pharmacotherapy should be used in conjunction with psychotherapy.
    d. Comorbid conditions should be treated with appropriate medications.
    e. Titration of medications should be slow.

17. Mothers of feeding-disorder infants are *least* likely to have which of the following?

    a. Repeated losses
    b. Severe depressions
    c. Hostile and angry interactions with their infants
    d. Enmeshed relationship with their own mothers
    e. Poverty

18. All of the following are characteristics of rumination disorder of infancy *except:*

    a. Regurgitation and rechewing of food
    b. Depressed appearance when ruminating
    c. Nonexistence of reliable data regarding its prevalence rates
    d. Poor regulation of an internal state of satisfaction
    e. A learned association and reinforcement

19. All of the following are common characteristics of pica *except:*

    a. Persistent eating of nonnutritive substances
    b. Cultural variations
    c. Medical complications such as heavy-metal poisoning
    d. Multifactorial etiology
    e. Association with anorexia nervosa

20. Compared to patients with restricting anorexia nervosa, patients with bulimia nervosa are more likely to have all of the following *except:*

    a. Depression
    b. High impulsivity
    c. Lack of control
    d. Low body weight (body mass index [BMI] < 17.5)
    e. Binge-eating behavior

21. Which of the following medical complications associated with anorexia nervosa is *least* likely to occur:

    a. Bradycardia
    b. Increased blood urea nitrogen (BUN)
    c. Leukocytosis
    d. Elevated liver enzymes and amylase
    e. Reduced bone mineral density

22. Which of the following is *least* likely to be a personality characteristic of patients with anorexia nervosa:

    a. Perfectionism
    b. Competitiveness
    c. Sense of responsibility
    d. Obsessional traits
    e. Interpersonal security

23. All of the following statements regarding the neuroendocrine etiological factors of anorexia nervosa are correct *except:*

    a. Serotonergic dysfunction may be related to both anorexia and bulimia.
    b. Both serotonin agonists and antagonists can be useful as adjunct treatments of anorexia nervosa.
    c. Cyproheptadine is helpful for bulimic patients.
    d. Low CSF 5-hydroxyindoleacetic acid level is found in bulimic patients.
    e. Low level of leptin is found in emaciated anorexic patients.

24. All of the following statements regarding the epidemiology of anorexia nervosa and bulimia nervosa accurately reflect current knowledge *except:*

    a. 90 to 95% are female.

b. Anorexia nervosa is more common than bulimia nervosa.

c. Anorexia nervosa is prevalent across different ethnic and socioeconomic groups.

d. There was a worldwide increase in incidence and prevalence rates of bulimia nervosa in the past decade.

e. There is ethnic variation in feeling pressure to be thin.

25. All of the following characterize families of girls with anorexia nervosa *except:*

a. The girl with anorexia nervosa is characterized as the symptom bearer of the family.

b. Her symptoms stabilize the family.

c. Mothers in families with a daughter with anorexia nervosa are characterized as overprotective.

d. These families are often described as disengaged.

e. Parents in these families can be both extremely nurturing and neglectful.

26. All of the following biologic factors are found in patients with anorexia nervosa *except:*

a. An association with a family history of mood disorders

b. Changes in neurotransmitter systems (noradrenergic, serotonergic, dopaminergic, and opioid)

c. Higher concordance for monozygotic as compared with dizygotic twins

d. Abnormal taste profiles

e. A responsible gene on chromosome 1p

27. All of the following statements regarding the long-term prognosis for anorexia nervosa accurately reflect current studies *except:*

a. Approximately 75% of patients improve or partially improve.

b. Approximately one fourth of patients become chronically ill.

c. Suicide attempts are rare (<10%).

d. The mortality rate at 10 years is approximately 5 to 7%.

e. Onset age between 12 and 18 years predicts a better prognosis than earlier or later onset.

28. Physical findings associated with bulimia nervosa include all of the following *except:*

a. Salivary-gland hypertrophy

b. Dental-enamel erosion

c. Poor skin turgor

d. Oliguria

e. Sluggish tendon reflex

29. All of the following are social–cultural influences on the development of anorexia nervosa *except:*

a. An association with "femininity"

b. Western culture's focus on thinness

c. Sparseness of food

d. Gender differences in socialization

e. Pressures for cultural assimilation by immigrants

30. All of the following statements regarding childhood obesity reflect current knowledge *except:*

a. Obesity in infancy does not necessarily predict obesity in childhood.

b. Obesity in childhood is a better predictor of later obesity than is obesity in infancy.

c. Fat-cell proliferation during infancy is the major determinant of the number of fat cells.

d. Approximately 60% of overweight 5-year-old children were overweight as infants.

e. A causal relationship is found between obesity and socioeconomic status.

31. All of the following statements regarding familial contributions to obesity are accurate *except:*

a. Overweight in parents is strongly correlated with overweight in their infants.

b. Overweight in parents is correlated with overweight in their children.

c. If one spouse is overweight, there is a 30% chance that the other spouse will be overweight too.

d. Twin and adoption studies support a strong genetic component to childhood obesity.

e. Children have a higher risk for overweight if both their parents are overweight than if only one parent is.

32. Which of the following genetic syndromes is *least* likely to cause obesity?

a. Prader–Willi syndrome

b. Cornelia de Lange's syndrome

c. Klinefelter's syndrome

d. Lawrence–Moon syndrome

e. Kleine–Levin syndrome

33. All of the following are characteristics of exogenous obesity in children *except:*

a. Excessive caloric intake

b. Genetic-familial factors

c. Familial disorganization

d. Height above the fifth percentile

e. Advanced bone age

ANSWERS AND EXPLANATIONS

1. (b) Except for answer **(b)** (should be decreased T3), all the hormonal abnormalities listed, among others such as growth hormone, vasopressin, and testosterone (males), can be found in emaciated patients with AN. Luteinizing hormone may reflect immaturity in patients with AN and explains the associated amenorrhea. In addition, other laboratory findings may include anemia, leukopenia, hypercarotenemia, hypoproteinemia, hypercholesterolemia, low basal metabolic rate, and reduced bone density. *(Ref. 3, pp. 694–695)*

2. (b) The concept of "Feeding Disorder of Infancy or Early Childhood" had been controversial until the formal definition was given in the DSM-IV in 1994, replacing failure to thrive among some other terms previously used. Feeding disorder is characterized by failure to eat adequately with significant failure to gain weight or significant weight loss over at least 1 month, not accounted for by an associated gastrointestinal, medical, or mental condition, and occurring before 6 years of age. Chatoor and colleagues proposed three distinct feeding disorders, including feeding disorder of homeostasis, attachment, and separation, respectively. These were recently modified to feeding disorder of state regulation and feeding disorder of caregiver–infant reciprocity by the Task Force on Research Diagnostic Criteria: Infancy and Preschool. *(Ref. 1, pp. 639–642; Ref. 3, p. 686; Ref. 4, pp. 107–108)*

3. (c) Infantile anorexia nervosa, so called because of its similarities to later onset anorexia nervosa, has separation-related conflicts as its core issue. The mother or caregiver becomes engaged in a conflict over who will control the infant's feeding. *(Ref. 1, pp. 644–645)*

4. (c) Feeding problems are not uncommon in infancy and early childhood. Up to 25% of healthy young children experience eating problems with even higher rates (up to 80%) in children with developmental delays. *(Ref. 1, p. 639)*

5. (d) Based on some long-term follow-up studies, 39% of patients with anorexia nervosa develop bulimia symptoms during the course of their illness, and meet full criteria for bulimia nervosa. When the patient pursues weight loss only through dieting, her disorder is referred to as "restricting type" AN. When both binge-eating and purging behavior are present, the disorder is referred to as "Binge-eating/purging type" *(Ref. 1, pp. 672, 685)*

6. (a) Salivary-gland (especially parotids) enlargement is more commonly associated with the self-induced vomiting in bulimic patients associated with elevated serum amylase. Lanugo hair is downy-like hair, especially on the arms; hypercarotenemia refers to yellow-tinged skin resulting from increased carotene. Both are the result of starvation of anorexic patients. Hypercholesterolemia can be seen in emaciated anorexic patients as well. *(Ref. 1, pp. 680, 696; Ref. 2, p. 107; Ref. 3, pp. 694–695)*

7. (b) While all of the disorders listed can occur with AN, the most common comorbid disorder is depression, followed by anxiety disorders that often precede the onset of the eating disorder. *(Ref. 1, p. 674)*

8. (c) While establishing rapport and stabilizing the family are important, the most important first step in the treatment of AN is nutritional restoration. Inpatient hospitalization may be necessary to achieve this goal, but at times it can be achieved in less restrictive settings. Once weight is brought to a medically stable level, the patient may be more amenable to more psychological treatments, and symptoms of obsessional thinking and mood and personality disturbance may improve. In general, patients respond best to a multifaceted treatment strategy with involvement of medical rehabilitation, individual cognitive therapy, group therapy, pharmacotherapy, and family therapy. *(Ref. 1, pp. 679–685; Ref. 2, pp. 109–112; Ref. 3, p. 697)*

9. (a) Resumption of normal physical and sexual development are used for premenarchal girls while 90% ideal body weight is used as a minimum target weight for patients with continuous menstruation at low body weights. The relationships between healthy body weight and published tables or the patient's or the family's ideal body weight are quite variable. Restoration of menses and ovulation is recommended as a healthy target weight by the American Psychiatric Association Work Group on Eating Disorders, 2000. *(Ref. 1, 681; Ref. 2, pp. 109–111)*

10. (d) The peak time of onset of BN is late adolescence or early adulthood, although the bulimia symptoms may be preceded by symptoms of anorexia nervosa at earlier ages. Based on numerous prevalence studies, the prevalence rate of BN in adolescent and young adult women is 1%, with a female to male ratio of 20:1 to 10:1. *(Ref. 3, p. 694; Ref. 4, p. 593)*

11. (e) Patients with Prader–Willi syndrome are not only usually hyperphagic but also obese, frequently accompanied by low IQ and hypotonia, which are not signs of AN. Crohn's disease and colitis can present with symptoms resembling those of anorexia nervosa, and the laxative-abusing bulimia patient may also have similar symptoms. Other physical disorders, such as diabetes mellitus, thyroid disease, acid peptic disease, intestinal motility disorder, and Addison's disease can all mimic symptoms of AN. *(Ref. 1, pp. 227, 675; Ref. 3, pp. 696–697)*

12. (a) Occasionally, higher rates have been reported, which reflect cultural or educational practices at the time, such as the belief that an infant cannot be overfed. *(Ref. 1, p. 661; Ref. 3, p. 687)*

13. (a) Obesity in females is nine times more common in social classes III and IV than in social classes I and II. Remember the saying, "You can never be too rich or too thin." A causal relationship between socioeconomic status and obesity has been proposed. Reports indicate that between 1983 and

1995, the prevalence rate of obesity among low-income preschool children in the United States increased consistently. The prevalence of overweight is higher in girls, with overall higher prevalence rate in Hispanic preschoolers. *(Ref. 1, pp. 661–662)*

14. **(e)** The respiratory hypoventilation and daytime hypersomnolence associated with the pickwickian syndrome and severe obesity have a reported mortality rate of 40%. Clinicians should also evaluate other potential comorbid conditions, complications, and preceding conditions that are associated with the obesity, such as slipper femoral epiphysis, cardiomegaly, hypoxia, hypertension, diabetes mellitus, papilledema, pneumonia, and polycythemia. *(Ref. 1, pp. 665–666)*

15. **(d)** Long-term follow-up studies show that 12 to 14% of patients with AN have a chronic course, with an approximate 34% remission rate, and 40% relapse rate. Mortality of women with AN is 12 times higher compared to the general population, with low serum albumin level, low body weight, poor social functioning, comorbid substance abuse/affective disorders, and longer duration of symptoms being the most important risk factors. The relationship between age of onset and outcome of AN is controversial, although late onset among other factors, such as comorbid with cluster B personality disorders/substance abuse and longer duration of symptoms, predicts a poorer outcome for BN. *(Ref. 1, pp. 684–685, 702)*

16. **(a)** Pharmacotherapy in treating anorexic adolescents should be combined with other psychosocial interventions. Fluoxetine did not show better treatment outcome in inpatient settings. However, for weight-recovered anorexic patients SSRIs seem to help maintain weight. Target symptoms should be identified when considering medications; the same principle applies to treatment of comorbid conditions. A low initiation dose and slow titration help to avoid potential side effects. *(Ref. 1, pp. 683–684)*

17. **(d)** The usual characteristics of mothers of infants who fail to thrive relate to an inability to nurture their infants based on a lack of nurturing in their own infancy and childhood and/or the lack of a satisfying relationship with another person. They may also experience repeated losses, acute and severe depression, and being angry and hostile toward their infants. They are more likely to be victims of abuse and domestic violence with higher rates of poverty and unemployment. Infants often attach to them insecurely. They tend to reject their children just like their parents rejected them when they were infants. *(Ref. 1, pp. 642–643)*

18. **(b)** In rumination disorder, the infant self-stimulates while ruminating and appears relieved and happy. The infant usually appears apathetic, withdrawn, or irritable when not ruminating. Infants with rumination seem to have poor capacity to regulate their internal state of satisfaction, and reinforcement and learned association develop between regurgitation and self-soothing. No epidemiological data of its prevalence or incidence rates are established. The role of genetic influence is unknown. Although according to the DSM-IV-TR criteria it cannot be due to an associated GI problem or other medical condition, it might be associated with gastroesophageal reflux disorder (GERD), and therefore medical evaluation is important in addition to psychiatric and behavioral assessment. Behavioral approaches and parent training are important parts of treatment among other modalities depending on the severity of the condition. Hospitalization may be necessary for some cases such as serious malnutrition. *(Ref. 2, pp. 73–75; Ref. 3, pp. 682–683; Ref. 4, pp. 105–106)*

19. **(e)** Infants and toddlers with pica will eat paint, plaster, hair, plants, paper, or sand, to name a few of the more common possibilities. As a result, these children can develop lead poisoning and bezoar (a ball of hair, paint, or other materials lodged in the intestinal tract). Pica is commonly associated with mental retardation, developmental delay, or severe deprivations. In some countries or particularly deprived areas, pica may be considered as normal in the culture, and may occur more commonly. It has a multifactorial etiology, and recent reports found possible association between pica and bulimia nervosa, not anorexia nervosa. *(Ref. 1, pp. 652–654; Ref. 2, pp. 71–73)*

20. **(d)** Bulimia nervosa patients are more distressed, depressed, and impulse disordered, with the sense of lack of control. Bulimia symptoms can precede or follow anorexia nervosa. Binge eating is one of the key criteria of bulimia, with vomiting being considered as a hallmark symptom. Patients with bulimia usually have normal body weight. Less than 85% of expected body weight or BMI < 17.5 is a key diagnostic criterion of anorexia nervosa. *(Ref. 1, pp. 679, 699; Ref. 2, p. 113; Ref. 4, pp. 589–594)*

21. **(c)** Cardiovascular complications associated with anorexia nervosa include hypotension, arrhythmia, bradycardia, and cardiac failure and arrest. Hematologic abnormalities include leukopenia (not leukocytosis), thrombocytopenia, and anemia. Gastrointestinal abnormalities include decreased gastric motility and emptying. Renal complications are the result of dehydration and decreased perfusion of the kidney and include elevated BUN, edema, and polyuria. Endocrine complications include amenorrhea and hypothyroidism, among others. Skeletal complications are the result of osteopenia and can cause broken bones. *(Ref. 1, pp. 672–674; Ref. 2, pp. 107–108)*

22. **(e)** In addition to interpersonal insecurity (not security) among other characteristics listed, minimization of emotional expression, identity confusion, rigid control over impulse, heightened industriousness, and underlying low self-esteem are all personality characteristics of the adolescents with AN. *(Ref. 1, p. 674)*

23. **(c)** Stress secondary to dieting and abnormal eating behaviors together with dysfunctions of endocrine and metabolic mechanisms may contribute to the development of eating disorders. An impaired serotonin neurotransmitter system, as well as dysfunction of the dopaminergic system, is associated with eating disorders. Adjunct treatments for anorexia nervosa can include serotonin agonists and antagonists, and cyproheptadine, a serotonin antagonist, is found to be helpful in gaining weight for anorexic restricting-type patients. Lower levels of CSF 5-hydroxyindoleacetic acid are found in patients with bulimia, whereas low levels of leptin are found in emaciated patients with anorexia. *(Ref. 3, p. 696)*

24. **(b)** Females have approximately 10 times higher prevalence and incidence rates of anorexia nervosa than males, with anorexia being less common than bulimia. There is rapid growth in the incidence and prevalence of bulimia based on epidemiological studies since 1990. In contrast to the old data that indicated anorexia was a typical illness in White and middle to upper-middle classes, more recent data suggest it is prevalent across different ethnic and socioeconomic groups. Racial differences are found in pressure on women to be thin, with Black women reporting less pressure than Whites. *(Ref. 1, pp. 675, 691–692)*

25. **(d)** Family dynamics in the case of anorexics are usually characterized by enmeshment rather than disengagement. On the other hand, some bulimic families are characterized as enmeshed, while others are characterized as disengaged. Families with anorexia nervosa are also described as rigid and mistrustful, and as lacking conflict resolution. The daughter's symptoms serve to divert attention from family conflict. *(Ref. 1, pp. 677–678, 695; Ref. 3, p. 696)*

26. **(e)** Based on family studies, the first- and second-degree relatives of patients with anorexia nervosa have higher risk for mood disorders. The changes in norepinephrine, serotonin, dopamine, and opioid neurotransmitter systems usually can be explained on the basis of weight loss rather than some factor specific to anorexia nervosa. Higher concordance rates in monozygotic twins of restricting anorexic patients support genetic etiology, although no genes have yet been identified. However, an anorexia nervosa susceptibility locus on chromosome 1p was identified based on a recent multisite genetic study. *(Ref. 1, pp. 678–679; Ref. 3, pp. 695–696)*

27. **(c)** Approximately 75% of anorexia nervosa patients are found to be improved or partially improved at 10-year follow-up, with one fourth of patients remaining chronically ill. Suicide attempts have been found to have been made by up to 24% of patients on follow-up. Mortality rate at 10-year follow-up is approximately 6.6%, and between 18 and 20% at 30-year follow-up. Onset before age 12 and after age 18 predicts a worse outcome than for the group with age of onset between 12 and 18 years. *(Ref. 1, pp. 684–685; Ref. 3, p. 698)*

28. **(d)** Polyuria (not oliguria) is common in bulimic patients. Other physical symptoms include hypotension; bradycardia; edema; arrhythmias; and oral, esophageal, and gastric damage from vomiting and/or binge eating. *(Ref. 1, pp. 696–697)*

29. **(c)** Anorexia nervosa is more prevalent in industrialized societies with Western cultural values, such as thinness and "femininity," and an abundance of food. Socialization pressures on girls may result in more pressure and anxiety resulting in simple solutions such as being thin. Immigrating to industrialized countries, immigrants may try to quickly assimilate the mainstream cultural value of "thinness equals success" and become more likely to develop eating disorders. *(Ref. 1, p. 678; Ref. 3, p. 695; Ref. 4, p. 587)*

30. **(c)** Obesity in infancy is a poor predictor of later obesity, although approximately 60% of obese 5-year-olds were obese in infancy. Fat-cell proliferation is more likely based on the degree and duration of the obesity, while the increase of fat cell size accounts for almost all the increase in fat storage during infancy. Socioeconomic status is also causally linked to obesity. *(Ref. 1, pp. 661–662)*

31. **(a)** Overweight parents are not more likely to have overweight infants, although this becomes less and less the case as the child becomes older. Intergenerational psychosocial influence and genetic contribution are associated with childhood obesity. Where one spouse is fat, 30% of the other spouses will also be fat, arguing against purely genetic factors in childhood obesity. Overweight in both parents transmits more familial risk to their children than overweight in only one parent. *(Ref. 1, p. 662; Ref. 3, pp. 687–688)*

32. **(b)** In addition to the listed syndromes (except for Cornelia de Lange's), Turner's, Alström, Bardet–Biedl, Beckwith–Wiedemann, and Cohen syndromes all can cause obesity. Cornelia de Lange's syndrome can cause growth retardation, mental retardation, and microcephaly. *(Ref. 1, pp. 227, 663)*

33. **(b)** Endogenous obesity is associated with some genetic, endocrinological, and neurological syndromes. Psychogenic causes of obesity have been observed, such as sudden weight gain following a traumatic separation from the primary caregivers and as a result of being in poorly organized families in which the child's needs are not perceived or met. In contrast to endogenous obesity (with lower percentile in height and delayed bone age), children with exogenous obesity tend to have excessive caloric intake and have normal height and advanced bone age. *(Ref. 1, pp. 663–664; Ref. 3, p. 688)*

7
MOVEMENT DISORDERS

QUESTIONS

Directions: Select the best response for each of the questions 1–16.

1. All of the following factors regarding genetic factors in Tourette's disorder are accurate *except:*

a. The concordance rate is higher for monozygotic as compared with dizygotic twins.

b. The transmission pattern is consistent with autosomal recessive.

c. More than 60% of Tourette's disorder is familial in origin.

d. First-degree relatives are at a higher risk for developing tics.

e. There is a genetic relationship between Tourette's disorder and obsessive–compulsive disorder (OCD).

2. All of the following statements regarding Tourette's disorder accurately reflect the current knowledge about the symptoms of the disorder *except:*

a. The initial symptoms appear between 5 and 8 years of age.

b. Tics progress from simple to complex.

c. Vocal tics precede motor tics by 1 to 2 years.

d. The frequency of occurrence varies widely.

e. Tics markedly decrease during sleep.

3. The percentage of patients with Tourette's disorder who meet criteria for OCD in adulthood is approximately:

a. 5%

b. 10%

c. 20%

d. 30%

e. 40%

4. Which of the following brain structures is *most* implicated in the pathogenesis of Tourette's disorder?

a. Basal ganglia

b. Cerebellum

c. Prefrontal cortex

d. Sensory motor strip

e. Hippocampus

5. Coprolalia occurs in what percentage of patients with Tourette's disorder?

a. <10%

b. 20%

c. 50%

d. 70%

e. >90%

6. Which of the following pharmacologic agents is considered the *most* potentially problematic for treatment of the inatten-

tion, distractibility, and impulsiveness occasionally seen in the patient with Tourette's disorder?

a. Clonidine

b. Stimulants

c. Strattera

d. Tenex

e. Some tricyclic antidepressant (TCA) agents

7. All of the following accurately describe tic disorders *except:*

a. They involve stereotyped movements or sounds.

b. The symptoms may diminish during sleep and absorbing activities.

c. Frequency of symptoms varies by day, week, and month.

d. The symptoms cannot be suppressed or deferred.

e. Younger children may be not aware of or minimize the symptoms.

8. Which of the following diagnoses is *most* appropriately considered for tics such as blinking or throat clearing lasting less than 4 weeks?

a. Tic disorder, not otherwise specified (NOS)

b. Chronic motor tic disorder

c. Chronic vocal tic disorder

d. Transient tic disorder

e. Tourette's disorder

9. Based on DSM-IV-TR, all of the following statements regarding transient tic disorder are accurate *except:*

a. The disorder is common in prepubertal children.

b. It is usually limited in duration.

c. It is exacerbated by stress.

d. It is more common in girls.

e. It has an onset before the age of 18 years.

10. Which of the following disorders is *most* likely to be genetically associated with Tourette's disorder?

a. Alcoholism

b. Schizophrenia

c. Depressive disorders

d. OCD

e. Bipolar disorder

11. Symptoms/conditions that are often associated with Tourette's disorder include all of the following *except:*

a. Learning difficulties

b. Psychosis

c. Inattentiveness, lability, and impulsiveness

d. Obsessive–compulsive phenomena

e. Mood lability

12. Which of the following differential diagnoses for Tourette's disorder is *least* important to be considered?

    a. Huntington's chorea
    b. Postviral encephalitis
    c. Schizophrenia, paranoid type
    d. Wilson's disease
    e. Tardive dyskinesia

13. Which of the following neurotransmitters is *most* likely to be abnormal in Tourette's disorder?

    a. Serotonin
    b. Epinephrine
    c. Acetylcholine
    d. Dopamine
    e. Glutamate

14. Which of the following classes of medications is *most* likely to aggravate tics?

    a. Neuroleptics
    b. Alpha-adrenergic agonists
    c. Benzodiazepines
    d. Stimulants
    e. Antihistamines

15. Which of the following pharmacologic agents has the *least* evidence for benefit in the treatment of Tourette's disorder?

    a. Guanfacine
    b. Clozapine
    c. Risperidone
    d. Ziprasidone
    e. Olanzapine

16. Based on current research, all of the following statements are true regarding Sydenham's chorea (SC) and pediatric autoimmune neuropsychiatric disorder associated with streptococcal infection (PANDAS) *except:*

    a. Patients with SC may experience complex tics, OCD, and attention-deficit hyperactivity disorder (ADHD) symptoms.
    b. PANDAS is considered as a unique clinical entity.
    c. A postinfectious autoimmune mechanism accounts for 60% of Tourette's disorder.
    d. The mechanisms associating SC and PANDAS are unclear and controversial.
    e. Immunomodulatory treatments for PANDAS are promising.

ANSWERS AND EXPLANATIONS

1. **(b)** It is generally accepted that the transmission pattern of Tourette's disorder is an autosomal dominant, while some recent studies indicate a more complex mode of inheritance. Genetic factors play a significant role in developing Tourette's disorder, which has been supported by twin, family, and other genetic studies. Some OCD cases and tic disorders share a common genetic vulnerability. *(Ref. 1, pp. 714–715; Ref. 3, p. 737; Ref. 4, p. 113)*

2. **(c)** The onset of motor tics usually precedes that of vocal tics by 1–2 years. Most motor tics are usually simple, and with time progress to complex tics. When tic symptoms occur frequently and prominently, they are very damaging to the child's self-esteem. *(Ref. 1, pp. 711–712)*

3. **(e)** By adolescence, the OCD symptoms associated with Tourette's disorder can be more apparent, which is especially true for compulsions. By adulthood, 40% of Tourette's patients develop full-blown OCD, with a male predominance (having a tic-related OCD compared to a non-tic-related OCD). *(Ref. 1, p. 712)*

4. **(a)** Support for the involvement of the basal ganglia include the large amounts of dopamine found in the region, postmortem studies, and positron-emission tomography studies in adults with Tourette's disorder. *(Ref. 1, p. 715; Ref. 3, p. 737)*

5. **(a)** While coprolalia (obscene language), a complex vocal tic, is traditionally associated with Tourette's disorder, it only occurs in less than 10% of cases. It usually first appears in early adolescence, and tends to decrease with age. Copropraxia (obscene gestures), a complex motor tic, may appear later. *(Ref. 4, pp. 109, 111)*

6. **(b)** The use of stimulants to treat symptoms of attention-deficit hyperactivity disorder in children with tics is very controversial since stimulants are known to be associated with the onset of tics and may make them worse. A recent study indicates that methylphenidate alone or combined with clonidine does not increase tics over a short period of time during the trial. Long-term study is not available at this time. All of the other medications have other specific concerns associated with their usage. *(Ref. 1, p. 721; Ref. 2, pp. 81–82; Ref. 3, pp. 740–742)*

7. **(d)** Tics can be suppressed or deferred for brief periods and decrease during sleep. All tics are abrupt, purposeless, and recurrent, and can be exacerbated by stress. Younger children may not recognize or deny the symptoms. Patients may experience more tics (a paroxysm phenomenon) after they suppress the tics for a while. *(Ref. 1, pp. 711–712; Ref. 3, pp. 736–737; Ref. 4, pp. 108–113)*

8. **(a)** The common vocal tics often include coughs, sniffs, barks, throat clearing, and other noises made during expiration while common motor tics include blinking, nose wrinkling, neck jerking, and shoulder shrugging. They are frequently thought of in connection with Tourette's disorder, but they can occur with all tic disorders. If tics last less than 4 weeks, the only diagnosis that applies is tic disorder, NOS. *(Ref. 4, pp. 109–116)*

9. **(d)** All tic disorders predominate in boys, and are quite common in prepubertal children. Transient tic disorder is time limited (between 4 weeks and 12 months) and usually is mild and benign, causing no severe impairment in most cases. Stress, fatigue, and excitement can exacerbate tics with usually a fluctuating presentation. Onset of any tic disorder should be before the age of 18 years, except for tic disorder, NOS. *(Ref. 1, p. 710; Ref. 4, pp. 115–116)*

10. **(d)** While OCD is more prevalent in patients with Tourette's, their first-degree relatives are more likely to have OCD than the general population, which indicates OCD and Tourette's may share common genetic risk factors. Family studies show a higher risk in male first-degree relatives to develop tics and OCD than in female relatives. *(Ref. 1, pp. 714–715; Ref. 3, p. 737)*

11. **(b)** Psychosis is rarely associated with Tourette's disorder. Learning difficulties and symptoms of ADHD may precede the appearance of tics. Obsessive–compulsive phenomena generally first appear in adolescence, and full-blown OCD is seen in approximately 40% of adults with Tourette's disorder. *(Ref. 1, p. 712; Ref. 4, p. 112)*

12. **(c)** Myoclonus, choreoathetosis, dystonia, akathisia, and excessive startle reactions need to be considered in the differential diagnosis for Tourette's disorder. Some of these can occur in patients with schizophrenia, but not usually in paranoid type. Patients with schizophrenia, catatonic type, may exhibit echolalia, echopraxia, excessive motor activity, and peculiarities of voluntary movement. Repetitive and stereotypical behaviors in patients with pervasive developmental disorder (PDD) should be considered, as well. *(Ref. 1, p. 713; Ref. 4, p. 315)*

13. **(d)** The most compelling evidence for involvement of any of the neurotransmitters in Tourette's disorder is for dopamine. Most of the support for the neurotransmitter dysfunction in Tourette's disorder is based on pharmacologic response and some recent imaging studies. Neuroleptics that preferentially block dopamine D_2 receptors are effective in decreasing tics. Dopamine agonists make them worse. Clonidine, an alpha-2-adrenergic receptor blocker, also leads to improvement in some tics. Exogenous opioids may also be altered. Serotonin has not been directly implicated, but is altered in OCD, which is frequently associated with Tourette's disorder. *(Ref. 1, p. 716)*

14. **(d)** Stimulants and certain antidepressants that affect the dopaminergic neurons may aggravate tics, but it is not clear whether they are etiologic, hasten the onset, or are coincidental with the onset. Neuroleptics and α-adrenergic agonists can be helpful in managing tics. *(Ref. 1, pp. 719–721; Ref. 2, p. 77)*

15. (b) About 60 to 90% of patients with Tourette's disorder respond to haloperidol, fluphenazine, and/or pemozide. Alpha-adrenergic agonists, such as clonidine and guanfacine, are especially helpful in mild cases. Some atypical neuroleptics (such as ziprasidone, olanzapine, and risperidone, but not clozapine) are shown to be efficacious in some studies. *(Ref. 1, pp. 719–721)*

16. (c) Postinfectious autoimmune mechanisms may be associated with only 10 to 20% of Tourette's cases. All of the other statements regarding PANDAS and SC are correct based on current research. *(Ref. 3, pp. 739, 742)*

8

DISORDERS OF SOMATIC FUNCTION (SLEEP, ELIMINATION, PSYCHOSOMATIC, AND SOMATOFORM DISORDERS)

QUESTIONS

Directions: Select the best response for each of the questions 1–36.

1. All of the following are characteristics of neonatal sleep patterns *except:*
   a. Rapid-eye-movement (REM) sleep occupies 50% of total sleep time.
   b. Stage 4 sleep accounts for 20% of total sleep time.
   c. Sleep-cycle length is approximately 50 minutes.
   d. The REM and non-REM (NREM) sleep states alternate with each other.
   e. Sleep begins with an initial REM period.

2. By what age are infants able to sleep uninterrupted through the night, up to 8.5 hours?
   a. 3 weeks
   b. 9 weeks
   c. 16 weeks
   d. 30 weeks
   e. 48 weeks

3. What is the *most* common sleep problem during the second year of life?
   a. Night awakenings
   b Nightmares
   c. Night terrors
   d. Struggles around going to bed
   e. Sleep apnea

4. By what age are dreams usually first reported?
   a. 1 year
   b. 2 years
   c. 3 years
   d. 4 years
   e. 5 years

5. All of the following can be considered as parasomnias phenomena *except:*
   a. Sleep apnea
   b. Sleep terror disorder (pavor nocturnus)
   c. Sleep talking (somniloquy)
   d. Nightmare disorder (dream anxiety disorder)
   e. Sleepwalking disorder (somnambulism)

6. Characteristics of the NREM parasomnias include all of the following *except:*
   a. They occur at the end of NREM stage 4 sleep.
   b. They occur just prior to a transition to REM sleep.
   c. They begin in school-age children.
   d. The individual has amnesia for the event.
   e. They are seen more frequently in females.

7. Characteristics of sleep terror disorder (pavor nocturnus) include all of the following *except:*
   a. Medication is often necessary in the treatment.
   b. Onset is between age 4 and 12 years, most commonly in children 3 to 6 years of age.
   c. It usually stops by adolescence.
   d. Adult onset predicts a chronic course.
   e. Parental attempts at consoling the child are ineffective.

8. All of the following statements regarding sleepwalking disorder (somnambulism) are accurate *except:*
   a. It is common in children 6 to 16 years of age.
   b. It may share a common neurophysiologic substrate with night terrors.
   c. Sleepwalkers are in little danger of hurting themselves.
   d. Seizures need to be considered in the differential diagnosis.
   e. Sleepwalking increases when the child is very tired or stressed.

9. Which of the following conditions is usually thought of as the *most* distressing to children and their parents?
   a. Nocturnal enuresis
   b. Dream anxiety disorder
   c. Sleep terror disorder
   d. Sleepwalking disorder
   e. Sleep talking disorder

10. All of the following statements regarding narcolepsy accurately reflect current knowledge *except:*
   a. Attacks of REM sleep occur during wakefulness.
   b. The onset of narcolepsy is around puberty.
   c. Stimulant drugs are used in the treatment.
   d. The most common misdiagnosis is attention-deficit hyperactivity disorder (ADHD).
   e. The adolescent often feels disoriented and fatigued upon awakening.

11. Disorders that *most* commonly coexist with enuresis include all of the following *except:*
   a. Developmental delays
   b. Encopresis
   c. Anxiety disorders
   d. Temper tantrums
   e. Sleep terror disorder

12. All of the following statements regarding the enuresis or urine alarm system are accurate *except:*
   a. A 60 to 80% initial response is reported.
   b. Combination with reward contingencies decreases the relapse rate.

c. Success is not dependent on parental involvement.

d. It is the most effective treatment for primary enuresis.

e. Explanations of its success are based on behavioral theories.

13. All of the following statements regarding encopresis are accurate *except:*

a. Prevalence is greater than 1% for boys.

b. Encopresis does not usually resolve until adolescence.

c. The disorder is more common in boys.

d. The disorder is more common in lower socioeconomic classes.

e. Certain children with encopresis show neurodevelopmental symptoms.

14. Which one of the following reactions to hospitalization is *most* characteristic of children 3 to 5 years of age?

a. Being upset by the change in routine

b. Having concerns about the loss of autonomy

c. Having compliance problems

d. Cause and effect understanding of the need to be in the hospital

e. Being upset by the separation from caregivers

15. Which of the following statements regarding somatization in youth is *incorrect?*

a. It occurs more in older children and adolescents.

b. Girls report somatic symptoms more consistently than boys.

c. In prepubertal children, recurrent abdominal pain (RAP) and headaches are more common than they are in adolescents.

d. In early childhood, girls and boys report frequency of recurrent pain equally.

e. Boys report more conversion symptoms than girls.

16. All of the following statements regarding conversion disorder represent our current knowledge *except:*

a. It usually occurs after a significant psychosocial stressor.

b. It is characterized by a pattern of recurring, multiple, clinically significant somatic complaints.

c. Cultural factors contribute to the development of symptoms.

d. It is rare in young children.

e. In children under 10 it is usually limited to gait problems or seizures.

17. All of the following characterize children less than 2 years of age with sleep problems *except:*

a. Their sleep problems are related to the parents' degree of involvement.

b. They are usually put in their crib awake rather than asleep.

c. They have more behavior problems.

d. Their mothers are more likely to have an insecure attachment to them.

e. They use their parents as a sleep aid.

18. All of the following are characteristic activities that occur during REM sleep *except:*

a. Active metabolic processes

b. Muscle-tone inhibition

c. Synchronized slower frequency waveforms on the electroencephalogram

d. Dreaming

e. Active central nervous system

19. All of the followings are characteristics of REM–NREM sleep cycles *except:*

a. In adults, sleep typically begins with NREM sleep.

b. In infants, sleep typically begins with REM sleep.

c. In infants, approximately 50% of sleep is REM sleep.

d. In adults, the percentage of NREM sleep is greater later in the sleep cycle.

e. REM–NREM sleep cycles are shorter in infants than in adults.

20. According to DSM-IV-TR, all of the following are considered major categories of sleep disorders *except:*

a. Dyssomnias

b. Other sleep disorders (such as substance-induced sleep disorder)

c. Parasomnias

d. Circadian rhythm sleep disorder

e. Sleep disorder related to another mental disorder

21. All of the following are characteristics of breathing-related sleep disorder *except:*

a. It may include repeated cycles of loud snoring followed by an apneic period, resulting in a brief arousal from sleep.

b. It may present as failure to thrive in children.

c. Daytime sleepiness is common.

d. Central sleep apnea is characterized by an absence of respiratory drive.

e. It is more common in girls.

22. Which of the following medical conditions is *least* likely a cause of breathing-related sleep disorder in children?

a. Enlarged tonsils and/or adenoids

b. Gross obesity

c. Maxillofacial abnormalities

d. Hyperthyroidism

e. Hypertension

23. Sleep terror disorder can be differentiated from nightmare disorder by all of the following *except:*

a. Time of the episode after sleep onset

b. Age of onset

c. Alertness after the episode

d. Remembrance of the episode

e. Amount of physiologic arousal

24. Which of the following classes of sleep disorders *most* frequently affect adolescents?

a. Phase delay syndromes
b. Sleepwalking
c. Sleep terrors
d. Nightmare disorder
e. Sleep apnea

25. All of the following are characteristically seen in narcolepsy *except:*

a. Attacks of REM sleep during wakefulness
b. High involvement with the serotonin neurotransmitter system
c. Sleep paralysis
d. Hypnagogic or hypnopompic auditory or visual hallucinations
e. Cataplexy

26. All of the following statements regarding functional enuresis are accurate *except:*

a. 80% of enuresis in children is primary.
b. The untreated remission rate is 10 to 20% per year.
c. The adult prevalence of enuresis is 1%.
d. Enuresis is usually associated with psychopathology.
e. Attention-deficit hyperactivity disorder, anxiety disorder, encopresis, and developmental delay can be commonly associated with enuresis.

27. Secondary enuresis may be related to all of the following *except:*

a. Geographic moves
b. Hospitalization
c. Unconscious, psychodynamic symbolism
d. Birth of a sibling
e. Child abuse

28. All of the following statements regarding the etiology of primary enuresis are accurate *except:*

a. Primary enuresis represents a maturational delay.
b. Genetic factors may play a role.
c. Medical disorders may account for the enuresis.
d. Enuresis is a disorder of stage 4 sleep.
e. Excessive fluid intake may be associated with the problem.

29. Which of the following medical conditions is *least* likely a cause of enuresis in children?

a. Prostate hypertrophy
b. Diabetes mellitus
c. Seizure disorder
d. Congenital malformation of the genitourinary tract
e. Urinary-tract infection

30. Effective treatments for primary enuresis include all of the following *except:*

a. Evening fluid restriction
b. Dry bed training
c. Enuresis alarm

d. Anticholinergic agents
e. Desmopressin

31. All of the following statements regarding primary encopresis are accurate *except:*

a. Children must be over 4 years of age to receive the diagnosis.
b. Frequency must be more than once a month for 3 months.
c. It may be associated with anismus.
d. Children develop this condition after a period of fecal continence.
e. Constipation and overflow incontinence are very common.

32. Encopresis may result from all of the following *except:*

a. Overinvolvement of the father
b. Painful defecation
c. Inadequate or punitive toilet training
d. Constipation, impaction, or retention
e. Toilet-related fears

33. Which of the treatments of retentive encopresis is *least* likely to be effective?

a. Behavioral therapy
b. Tricyclic antidepressants (TCAs)
c. Diet modification
d. Disimpaction
e. Bowel retraining

34. All of the following suggestions are useful for a psychiatrist who is working with a family that resists psychiatric evaluation for the child's possible somatization disorders *except:*

a. Delay making a definite etiological diagnosis.
b. Gather detailed information focusing on psychosocial history, stress, and emotional consequences of the dysfunction.
c. Start the psychiatric evaluation after completing other workups.
d. Report to the state authority, if necessary, to avoid further needless invasive procedures.
e. Focus on dysfunction, not diagnosis.

35. Which of the following chronic medical diseases is *least* likely to be associated with psychological symptoms?

a. Seizure disorder
b. Diabetes
c. Cystic fibrosis
d. Inflammatory bowel disease
e. Hypotension

36. All of the following tests are commonly used as a part of psychological evaluation of a child with a physical illness *except:*

a. The eating attitude test
b. The high-sensitivity cognitive screen
c. Rorschach Inkblot
d. The coping health inventory for parents
e. The Varni–Thompson Pediatric Pain Questionnaire

ANSWERS AND EXPLANATIONS

1. **(b)** In the neonate, stage 4 sleep does not take place. In contrast to neonates and infants, adults spend 20% of total sleep time in REM sleep and 80% in NREM sleep, and stages 3 and 4 sleep account for approximately 20% of NREM sleep. The length of sleep cycle in adults is approximately 90 minutes, which is longer than that of infants (50 minutes). *(Ref. 1, p. 728)*

2. **(c)** More frequent alternations between wakefulness and sleep occur in newborns, and diurnal wakefulness lengthens as infants age. The diurnal cycle usually establishes by the age of 5 weeks, and infants can sleep uninterrupted up to 8.5 hours by week 16. One early study also found 70% of infants can sleep through the night by the age of 3 months. However, video studies show that, at 6 months of age, infants' sleep is interrupted once or twice 5 to 6 hours into the sleep, and one third to half of those interruptions result in a return to sleep without crying. *(Ref. 1, p. 731; Ref. 3, p. 876)*

3. **(d)** It is common for children in their second year of life to resist bedtime. This may be due to separation anxiety or fears of the dark or being alone. Chronic childhood insomnia is more frequent in children with psychiatric disorders. *(Ref. 1, p. 732)*

4. **(c)** Dreams are usually first reported by age 3, followed by nightmares shortly after. Dream content is usually short and concrete before age 8. *(Ref. 1, p. 732)*

5. **(a)** Parasomnias are sleep disorders in which episodes of non-waking activity interrupt sleep suddenly and intermittently. Based on DSM-IV-TR, sleep talking is not listed as a separated sleep disorder, but it occurs in NREM stage 4 sleep, just like sleepwalking and night terror. Sleep apnea, on the other hand, is categorized under breathing-related sleep disorder, which is subgrouped into obstructive and central sleep apnea syndromes. *(Ref. 1, pp. 734–735; Ref. 4, pp. 615–616, 630–631)*

6. **(e)** The ratio of males to females is 6 to 8:1, and there is a strong positive family history of NREM stage 4 parasomnias along male lines. Parents of children with parasomnias are distressed over their occurrence, but the children are not aware of the episodes. Parasomnias were thought to occur only in NREM stage 4 sleep, but REM parasomnias (REM sleep behavior disorder) are said also to occur, although they are uncommon in children. *(Ref. 1, p. 734)*

7. **(a)** Children usually outgrow the disorder by adolescence. Medications are not usually indicated in the treatment of night terrors. Support, education, and patience while waiting for the child to outgrow the disorder are usually satisfactory. When more of an intervention is necessary, a low dose of benzodiazepine or imipramine can provide symptomatic relief. When the disorder begins in adulthood, it often has a chronic course. *(Ref. 1, p. 734; Ref. 2, pp. 165–167; Ref. 3, pp. 881–882; Ref. 4, pp. 634–636)*

8. **(c)** While sleepwalking, children are poorly coordinated and are not capable of complex behaviors. They are therefore in danger of hurting themselves. Seizure disorder needs to be considered in the differential diagnosis, especially when the disorder persists into adolescence. Maturational factors may play a role in both sleepwalking and sleep terror, and a common neurophysiologic substrate for both of the disorders has been suggested. *(Ref. 1, p. 735; Ref. 2, pp. 167–168; Ref. 3, pp. 881–882)*

9. **(a)** Sleep-related enuresis can occur primarily in REM stage, with the majority of episodes occurring during the first third of the night. The condition can have a long impact on the children and their parents, being thought of as the most distressing due to duration, compared to other sleep disorders in children. *(Ref. 3, pp. 882–883)*

10. **(e)** After an attack, the adolescent with narcolepsy feels refreshed, which contrasts with the excessive somnolence in other dyssomnias that can cause nonrestorative sleep. Adolescents with narcolepsy often fidget to ward off feelings of sleepiness, which leads to the misdiagnosis of ADHD. *(Ref. 1, pp. 736–737; Ref. 2, pp. 162–163; Ref. 3, pp. 878, 880)*

11. **(d)** No association has been established between enuresis and tics, biting, temper tantrums, fire setting, and cruelty to animals. Enuresis is occasionally associated with such psychiatric disorders as anxiety disorders, oppositional defiant disorder, and ADHD, and also commonly coexists with encopresis, some sleep disorders, and developmental delays. *(Ref. 1, p. 743; Ref. 2, p. 88; Ref. 4, p. 119)*

12. **(c)** Parents need to be involved to prevent relapse. The alarm system is a modification of the "bell and pad," and works best when the alarm awakens the parent, who then awakens the child to go to the bathroom. Effectiveness of the treatment is based on behavioral conditioning. Combining treatment with reward contingencies seems to decrease the relapse rate. *(Ref. 1, p. 745; Ref. 2, pp. 90–91; Ref. 3, pp. 702–703)*

13. **(b)** Encopresis is rarely seen after the age of 8. Higher rates are seen in children with moderate to severe mental retardation. *(Ref. 1, pp. 745–747; Ref. 2, pp. 82–83)*

14. **(e)** Infants are most upset by the change in routine. School-age children are beginning to have an understanding of the etiology of their illness, although irrational explanations of the illness still occur. Before then, children are likely to feel illness is a punishment for wrongdoing. Adolescents, in their struggle for autonomy, may be noncompliant. *(Ref. 1, pp. 755–756; Ref. 2, pp. 244–246; Ref. 3, pp. 1236–1237)*

15. **(e)** Somatization disorder is overall more prevalent in females than males. While recurrent somatic complaints occur in 11% of girls and 4% of boys between 12 and 16 years of age, only approximately 1% meet DSM diagnostic criteria for somatization disorder. Recent studies show older children and adolescents seem to have more somatic complaints, with girls

reporting symptoms in more consistent ways than boys. In younger children, recurrent abdominal pain and headaches are more prevalent symptoms, which occur with equal frequency in both genders. Girls across all ages report more conversion or pseudoneurological symptoms than boys. (Ref. 3, pp. 848–849; Ref. 4, pp. 486–488)

16. (b) Answer b is a definition of somatization disorder. When this diagnosis is made, the diagnosis of conversion disorder should not be made, although they can occur in the same individual. Conversion disorder is usually limited in the number of symptoms and the time course in contrast to somatization disorder, which tends to be chronic and involves multiple symptoms. (Ref. 3, pp. 849–850; Ref. 4, pp. 492–496)

17. (b) The more involved a parent becomes in the infant's sleep, the more likely that a sleep problem will develop. Infants who feed to sleep or who are put to bed asleep are more likely to wake at night and need to use their parents as a sleep aid to fall back to sleep rather than be able to self-soothe or use an inanimate object to help themselves fall back to sleep. Poor sleepers wake as often as normal sleepers but are more likely to have behavior problems, difficult temperament, and adverse medical histories, with their mothers feeling an insecure attachment to them. (Ref. 1, pp. 731–732; Ref. 3, pp. 878–879)

18. (c) Slow, high-voltage, synchronized delta waves occur during stages 3 and 4 of NREM sleep. Rapid-eye-movement sleep is characterized by neuronal firing, neurotransmitter turnover, and metabolic activities that resemble wakefulness. Mental activity also resembles wakefulness and is reported as dreams. Muscle-tone inhibition occurs in REM sleep. (Ref. 1, pp. 727–728; Ref. 3, p. 876)

19. (d) The majority of NREM sleep occurs in the early part of the sleep cycle in adults, with a higher proportion of REM found in infants. In infants, REM–NREM cycle length is approximately 50 minutes, in contrast to 90 minutes in adults. Infants spend approximately 50% of sleep in REM sleep. During maturation, the prominence of REM sleep decreases. (Ref. 1, p. 728; Ref. 3, pp. 876–877)

20. (d) Circadian rhythm sleep disorder (formerly sleep-cycle disorder) is subcategorized under the major category of dyssomnias according to DSM-IV-TR. Dyssomnias are disorders of initiating and maintaining sleep such as insomnia. Parasomnias are unusual sleep-related behaviors and events. (Ref. 4, pp. 597–661)

21. (e) Obstructive sleep apnea, the most common form of breathing-related sleep disorder, is characterized by peripheral obstruction of the airway while central sleep apnea is characterized by a lack of respiratory drive. Daytime sleepiness is the result of repeated awakenings, which can also result in failure to grow, and behavioral and attention problems. Breathing-related sleep disorders are more prevalent in males. (Ref. 3, pp. 880–881; Ref. 4, pp. 615–622)

22. (d) Gross obesity associated with the pickwickian syndrome is a serious cause of sleep apnea. Other causes include systemic hypertension, lax upper-airway structures, gastroesophageal reflux, and dysfunction of the central control of breathing. Hypothyroidism (not hyperthyroidism) is also associated with

sleep apnea. (Ref. 2, pp. 163–164; Ref. 3, p. 881; Ref. 4, pp. 618–619)

23. (b) Night terror disorder occurs 90 to 120 minutes after the onset of sleep. Children are difficult to arouse from an episode and often appear terrified and inconsolable, and they have no or little memory of the episode. Nightmare disorder, on the other hand, takes place in the latter half of the sleep cycle. Children are usually easily arousable and consolable, and they are alert afterward, with memory of the dream. Both disorders can have an onset during young childhood; therefore, it is difficult to differentiate one from the other by using the age of onset. (Ref. 3, pp. 882–883; Ref. 4, pp. 631–638)

24. (a) Phase delay occurs when the circadian rhythm becomes delayed as the adolescent stays up later and later at night and then sleeps late in the morning. In DSM-IV-TR it is called circadian rhythm sleep disorder. Narcolepsy is the disorder of excessive somnolence that begins in adolescence, and sleepiness is the most frequent initial complaint. These two conditions commonly affect adolescents, while other listed conditions more commonly affect younger children. (Ref. 1, pp. 736–737; Ref. 4, pp. 609–614, 622–628)

25. (b) In narcolepsy, REM sleep attacks interrupt the waking state and lead to all of the symptoms listed, except for answer b. Instead, dysfunction of cholinergic–dopaminergic interaction has been proposed. Cataplexic attacks are often preceded by intense emotional outbursts. Recent genetic studies show genetic factors play important roles in the etiology of narcolepsy, supported by presence of certain HLA alleles that are more prevalent in patients with narcolepsy than in the general population. With a recent discovery of a narcolepsy gene in dogs, active searching for human narcolepsy gene(s) is being undertaken. (Ref. 1, pp. 736–737; Ref. 2, pp. 162–163; Ref. 4, pp. 609–614)

26. (d) Most children with enuresis do not have a coexisting psychiatric disorder, although some common conditions listed in answer e can be comorbid with enuresis. Primary enuresis occurs in children who are not bladder trained. (Ref. 1, p. 743; Ref. 2, pp. 86–87)

27. (c) Secondary enuresis refers to urinary incontinence that takes place after a period of continence of at least 1 year. It is related to stress, trauma, or psychosocial crisis, with no evidence to support the presence of a symbolic meaning. (Ref. 1, p. 744)

28. (d) Enuresis has not been found to be associated with a particular stage of sleep. Genetic and family studies show a genetic contribution to enuresis, with a higher monozygotic concordance rate and approximately 70% of probands having a first-degree relative with functional enuresis, especially in the case of boys. Since no single cause of enuresis has been identified, a multifactorial theory still prevails. (Ref. 1, p. 744; Ref. 2, pp. 87–88; Ref. 3, pp. 882–883)

29. (a) Prostate hypertrophy is not a common cause of enuresis in children. More common medical causes include diabetes insipidus, urethritis, sickle cell trait, neurogenic bladder, urinary obstruction, renal insufficiency, and neuroleptic-induced

enuresis. Urinary-tract infection is more commonly the cause in girls. *(Ref. 1, p. 744; Ref. 2, p. 89)*

30. **(d)** Stimulants, sedatives, and anticholinergic agents have not been found helpful. Since primary enuresis is primarily a benign and self-limited disorder, reassurance and support are usually sufficient with younger children. Tricyclic antidepressants and desmopressin are helpful symptomatically. Dry bed training techniques, such as retention-control training, positive-practice nighttime awakening, etc., can be helpful when used along with an alarm system. *(Ref. 1, p. 745; Ref. 2, pp. 90–91; Ref. 3, p. 883)*

31. **(d)** Encopresis is the repeated passage of feces into places inappropriate for that purpose, occurring after age 4 when bowel control is expected. Children with primary encopresis have never developed fecal continence. Constipation and overflow incontinence can be associated with both primary and secondary encopresis, with anismus present in 75% of encopresis cases. *(Ref. 1, pp. 746–747; Ref. 2, pp. 82–84; Ref. 3, pp. 706–707; Ref. 4, pp. 116–118)*

32. **(a)** No single pathophysiologic or psychodynamic explanation accounts for the etiology of encopresis. Individual and family psychopathology are more common in children with functional encopresis than in the general population. An uninvolved, passive father and a domineering mother with ambivalence towards the child's autonomy are associated with encopresis. *(Ref. 1, p. 747; Ref. 2, pp. 83–84; Ref. 3, p. 706)*

33. **(b)** While some TCAs (imipramine and amitriptyline) have shown symptom improvements in nonretentive encopresis, TCAs are contraindicated for retentive encopresis. For children with severe stool retention, bowel impaction, or loss of bowel tone, an initial bowel cleanout followed by bowel retraining is necessary. Education and increased fiber and water in the diet are also useful. *(Ref. 1, pp. 747–748; Ref. 2, pp. 85–86; Ref. 3, p. 707)*

34. **(c)** Child psychiatric evaluation should be initiated from the beginning, especially if the child needs pediatric hospitalization. In suggesting a referral for psychiatric evaluation, it is important that the treating physician agrees with the referral and that the family be adequately informed about the referral request by the treating physician. Sometimes, families resist psychiatric evaluations. *(Ref. 1, pp. 758–759)*

35. **(e)** Alexander's original study of psychosomatic disorders included asthma, peptic ulcer, rheumatoid arthritis, ulcerative colitis, neurodermatitis, thyrotoxicosis, and essential hypertension. Also included is anorexia nervosa. Children and adolescents with chronic illness without disability are reported to be twice as likely to have a psychiatric disorder as are normal controls. *(Ref. 1, pp. 751, 754–755)*

36. **(c)** All the questionnaires and tests listed, except for the Rorschach Inkblot, were developed and are commonly used to assess children and families with physical problems thought to be related to psychological factors. Projective tests have not been used generally to identify psychological factors in somatic disorders. *(Ref. 1, pp. 757–758)*

9

SUBSTANCE USE AND ABUSE

QUESTIONS

Directions: Select the best response for each of the questions 1–20.

1. All of the following statements about the interaction between environmental and genetic/familial influences on alcoholism are true *except:*

   a. Adopted-away children of parents with alcoholism have increased risks of developing alcoholism.
   b. Adopted children whose adoptive parents are using alcohol do not have a higher risk of developing alcoholism.
   c. Early onset of heavy drinking is not associated with increased risk of the use of other substances.
   d. Alcoholism may be associated with the dopamine D_2 receptor gene marked by the A_1 allele.
   e. Children of parents with alcoholism have higher tolerance to alcohol.

2. All of the following epidemiology data regarding drug and alcohol use in adolescents are correct *except:*

   a. There was a decreased use of ecstasy in high school seniors between 1998 and 2001.
   b. Use of alcohol has been fairly stable.
   c. Compared to 1992, there was increased marijuana use in 2001.
   d. There is an increased use of anabolic steroids, with an almost double rate in 2001 compared to the rate in 1994.
   e. LSD use almost peaked again in high school seniors in 1997.

3. All of the following statements regarding the initiation and progression of drug use are accurate *except:*

   a. For most illicit drugs, if there is no abuse prior to age 20, it is less likely thereafter.
   b. Problematic drinking in adolescence is related to substance abuse in adulthood.
   c. The age of first use of marijuana has been decreasing in recent years.
   d. Most substance use progresses in generally predictable stages.
   e. Most youth who experiment with alcohol and illicit drugs will progress to alcoholism and substance abuse.

4. All of the following statements regarding the association of family characteristics with substance abuse in youth are accurate *except:*

   a. Combining multiple risk factors may influence continued drug use.
   b. Lack of parental monitoring is associated with initiation of illicit drug use in younger children (<11 years of age).
   c. Children with parents who smoke are more likely to initiate smoking through a modeling mechanism.

   d. Family abuse increases substance abuse only in the families with substance abuse.
   e. Children from a family without discipline, praise, or positive family relationships are more likely to abuse illicit drugs.

5. All of the following cultural and societal factors are associated with drug use *except:*

   a. Laws favorable to drug use
   b. Social norms favorable to drug use
   c. Affluent economic status
   d. Availability of substances
   e. Neighborhood disorganization

6. All of the following statements regarding the use of a urine drug screen in the evaluation and monitoring of potential substance abuse in young people are correct *except:*

   a. Collection of urine samples must be under observation.
   b. Very few drug-using teens know how to adulterate urine samples.
   c. Testing results can be altered by adding a small amount of bleach or diluting the urine.
   d. Tests can detect the presence of different drugs in urine samples only within certain time frames.
   e. Marijuana can be detected in urine samples for up to 1 month in chronic users.

7. All of the following statements regarding the successful treatment of substance abuse in youth are accurate *except:*

   a. It usually begins with medical detoxification.
   b. Abstinence is important.
   c. Use of self-help groups such as Alcoholics Anonymous can be helpful.
   d. The concept of "recovery" is utilized rather than that of cure.
   e. Group therapy with other adolescent abusers is employed.

8. All of the following characteristics of substance abuse in adolescents compared to adults are true *except:*

   a. Adolescents are less likely to have associated health conditions than adults.
   b. Life-threatening withdrawal symptoms can occur.
   c. Inpatient detoxification may be necessary.
   d. Adolescents tend to be more open about their drug use (amount, type, frequency, etc.)
   e. Inpatient psychiatric care may be due to danger to self or others, and psychotic symptoms.

9. The most likely outcome of substance abuse among children and adolescents is:

   a. Progression to chemical dependency

b. Casual use without significant consequences
c. Significantly more psychiatric problems
d. Increased unemployment
e. Increased trouble with the law

10. Which of the following conditions is *least* likely to be comorbid with a substance use disorder?

a. Depression
b. Bipolar disorder
c. Anxiety disorder
d. Attention-deficit hyperactivity disorder (ADHD)
e. Anorexia nervosa, restricting type

11. Intensive outpatient and partial hospital programs are suitable for which of the following stages of substance use:

a. Experimental use
b. Regular use
c. Preoccupation with use
d. Chemical dependence
e. Chemical intoxication and risk of withdrawal seizure

12. All of the following neuropsychological traits are associated with developing substance use disorders *except*:

a. Impulsivity
b. Behavioral overactivity and aggression
c. Sensation seeking
d. High sociability and obedience
e. Peer rejection

13. All of the following are characteristics of type 2 or type B alcoholism proposed by Cloninger and Babor, respectively, *except*:

a. High genetic loading for alcoholism and substance abuse
b. A late onset of drinking behaviors
c. Deviant behaviors
d. High novelty seeking
e. Low harm avoidance

14. All of the following are often found in youth who are acutely intoxicated with opiates *except*:

a. Enlarged pupils
b. Drowsiness
c. Reduced cough reflex
d. Constipation
e. Nausea and vomiting

15. All of the following statements regarding inhalant or solvent abuse among young people are accurate *except*:

a. Inhalants and solvents are popular for abuse among economically disadvantaged populations.
b. Physiological effects may include excitation, depression, and disorientation.
c. Typical inhalants include volatile gases, toluene products, and halogenated hydrocarbons.
d. The effects are usually short-lived, with little long-term consequences.

e. Solvent abuse is associated with sudden sniffing death syndrome.

16. All of the following stages of change are suggested in motivational treatment *except*:

a. Precontemplation
b. Contemplation
c. Preparation
d. Recognition of higher power
e. Action

17. All of the following statements regarding dual diagnosis among adolescents are accurate *except*:

a. There is a strong association of substance and alcohol abuse with suicide attempts.
b. Substance abuse is not commonly found with eating disorders such as bulimia nervosa.
c. Patients with dual diagnosis have higher relapse rates.
d. Sexual abuse is associated with more frequent use of alcohol, marijuana, and stimulants, with earlier onset of use.
e. Posttraumatic stress disorder (PTSD) and depression are strongly associated with alcohol dependence in girls.

18. Which of the following general statements regarding substance abuse treatment for children and adolescents is *inaccurate*?

a. Levels of care should be determined based on the stage of substance involvement.
b. Family psychopathology and involvement in treatment are important predictors of outcome.
c. Multisystemic therapy assesses various systems, and changes the behavior and relationships based on the strengths and weaknesses of the multiple systems involved.
d. Cognitive–behavioral therapy (CBT) group therapy has a better short-term outcome than the interactional group.
e. Multisystemic therapy shows similar outcome compared to probation or counseling.

19. All of the following statements regarding substance use/abuse prevention programs are correct *except*:

a. Essential aspects of effective programs include program focus, delivery technique, evaluation and training, and support.
b. Programs with informational or affective components are more effective than those that use social influence and life skills approaches.
c. Effective programs include Project SMART, Life Skills Training, and Project STAR.
d. Programs using interactive techniques are more effective than those using noninteractive ones.
e. The Reconnecting Youth Program targets depression, substance use, and suicidal ideation, building resilience in youth with poor academic achievement.

20. Which of the following statements regarding pharmacological interventions related to substance use disorders and comorbid conditions in youth is *least* accurate?

a. Published research data are few.
b. Lithium decreases alcohol use in youth with bipolar disorder and secondary substance dependence.
c. Stimulants should not be used in youth with both ADHD and a substance use disorder.
d. Youth with ADHD, if treated, have lower risk of developing a substance abuse.
e. Fluoxetine shows effectiveness in treating drug-dependent delinquents with depression.

ANSWERS AND EXPLANATIONS

1. **(c)** Both genetic and environmental factors influence the development and progress of alcoholism and other substance use disorders. In general, the early onset of alcohol and substance use predicts poorer outcomes. The heavy drinking at an early age predicts a higher prevalence of use of other substances in the future. Adoptive studies suggest strong genetic influence on alcoholism. A recent study also shows that children of alcoholic parents have a higher tolerance for alcohol, needing a higher amount of alcohol to delay the reflex response. An association between the D_2 receptor (allele A_1 on chromosome 11) and alcoholism was found, although it has not been consistently replicated and may be nonspecific because A_1 is also associated with Tourette's disorder, ADHD, and autism. (*Ref. 3, pp. 896–897*)

2. **(a)** A club drug named flunitrazepam fell off as a favorite in recent years, whereas another club drug, ecstasy (MDMA), has become very popular among older teens. Among high school seniors, the lifetime prevalence for alcohol use has remained high for the past 25 years. Marijuana is the most frequently used illegal drug, with a decreased use in 1992 and an increase again in 2001. Recent increased use of anabolic steroids is concerning. LSD use showed another peak in seniors in 1997. (*Ref. 1, pp. 796–797; Ref. 2, p. 119*)

3. **(e)** Except for prescription drugs, most illicit drug abuse starts in adolescence. Problematic drinking in adolescence is an indicator of subsequent abuse. There is a recent trend towards a decreased age of onset for marijuana use. Most illicit drug abuse develops in predictable stages, with initiation of gateway substances followed by other and multiple drugs, which lead to abuse or dependence. However, most adolescents who experiment with alcohol and/or illicit drugs do not develop substance use disorders. (*Ref. 2, pp. 120–121; Ref. 3, pp. 895–897*)

4. **(d)** There are numerous risk and protective factors that lead towards substance abuse in youth or prevent it. Family influence is very important. Rarely, only one risk factor leads to substance abuse; with multiple factors interacting with one another, different combinations of risk and protective factors predict different outcomes. Parental modeling, parental submissive attitude towards drug use, family disruption, and the lack of discipline and positive relationships are significant risk factors. Family abuse is a risk factor either with or without a previous family history of substance abuse. (*Ref. 1, p. 800; Ref. 2, pp. 119–120; Ref. 3, pp. 896–897*)

5. **(c)** All the listed cultural and societal factors (except for answer **c**) are associated with substance use. Extreme economic deprivation (not affluent economic status) is also a risk factor. There are a variety of cultural and societal differences in attitudes towards substance use, patterns of use, accessibility of drugs, physical reactions to alcohol and drug usage, and even in laws that regulate substance use. (*Ref. 3, p. 896; Ref. 4, pp. 205, 219*)

6. **(b)** Urine drug screening is the most commonly used method to monitor and evaluate adolescent drug use. Urine samples are very easily adulterated, and most teens know how to beat the urine drug screen. Replacing a urine sample with apple juice, diluting it, or adding bleach or blood can all alter the test results, usually leading to a false negative finding. That is why collection of the urine sample should be under observation. There are limitations of urine drug screening, especially because different drugs can be detected in the urine for a certain amount of time after the most recent use, ranging from 1 day to 1 month, depending on the drug and how long it has been used. (*Ref. 3, p. 901*)

7. **(a)** Medical detoxification is rarely necessary for the majority of adolescent substance abusers. Family treatment is an essential part of successful treatment. Groups with other adolescents without adult abusers work better than mixed-age groups. (*Ref. 1, p. 805; Ref. 2, pp. 122–124; Ref. 3, pp. 901–906*)

8. **(d)** Adolescents may minimize their alcohol or drug use, which can be dangerous because they may experience severe withdrawal symptoms from some of the drugs, such as benzodiazepines and other sedatives. Even though adolescents may have better general health than adults, inpatient hospitalization may still be necessary for a full evaluation/stabilization, severe withdrawal (even though it is relatively rare), psychosis, and high-risk behaviors, such as danger to self or others. (*Ref. 1, p. 805; Ref. 3, p. 905*)

9. **(b)** While all of the outcomes listed are possible, only a small number of those individuals will develop true substance abuse or dependence, usually leading to some impairments and complications. (*Ref. 2, p. 121; Ref. 4, pp. 205–206*)

10. **(e)** A comorbid psychiatric disorder with a substance use disorder is referred to as a "dual diagnosis." Adolescents and adults with substance use disorders have a higher chance than the general population of having another psychiatric condition, with depression and other mood disorders, anxiety disorders, oppositional defiant disorder, conduct disorder, antisocial personality disorder, ADHD, schizophrenia, and bulimia among the more common ones. It is often difficult to distinguish whether substance use disorder is the primary or secondary disorder. Therefore, careful assessment and evaluation for a possible dual diagnosis and appropriate treatments for both disorders are important. (*Ref. 1, pp. 805–808; Ref. 2, p. 119*)

11. **(c)** Cognitive behavioral treatment, 12-step programs, and intensive outpatient and partial programs can be used appropriately during the stage of preoccupation with use. More or less restrictive settings (levels of care) can be used for other stages of use. (*Ref. 1, pp. 800–805*)

12. **(d)** Aggressive behavior is shown to predict heavy substance abuse in adolescence, particularly for males. Substance-abusing adolescents can be discriminated from normal controls on a variety of temperamental scales closely linked to

behavioral-activity regulation. Sensation seeking is a person-ality trait defined by the need for novel and complex sensations and experiences and a willingness to undergo risks to have such experiences. A strong connection is found to exist between sensation seeking and drug use. Impulsivity, rebelliousness (not obedience), and peer rejection (not high sociability) are also among the risk factors for developing substance use disor-ders. *(Ref. 1, p. 800; Ref. 2, p. 120; Ref. 3, pp. 896–897)*

13. (b) Cloninger and Babor have proposed a classification scheme whereby a subgroup of patients with a high genetic loading for alcoholism/substance abuse, an early onset of alcoholism, a rapid and severe course, deviant behaviors, and coexisting psychological problems are classified as type 2 or type B alco-holism. They also share some temperament traits found under Newcomb's psychobehavioral factors. Cloninger's type 1 and Babor's type A alcoholism show opposite characteristics of those mentioned here. *(Ref. 3, p. 897)*

14. (a) In an acute opiate intoxication state, miosis (pinpoint pupils, not enlarged pupils), among other physiological effects such as drowsiness, nausea/vomiting, decreased cough reflex, hypothermia, hypotension, bradycardia, and respiratory/cen-tral nervous system depression, can be seen. Overdose can occur, especially when opiates are combined with alcohol and other sedatives, and may lead to death. *(Ref. 3, p. 899)*

15. (d) The effects of solvent abuse can be grave, with permanent and irreversible damage to the brain (especially the frontal lobes and cerebellum), and possible demyelination, causing hearing loss, peripheral neuropathy, liver and kidney damage, and leukemia. Volatile gases include gasoline and butane; tol-uene products include glues, acrylic paints, paint thinners, and automotive products; and halogenated hydrocarbons include freon, solvents, spot removers, and typewriter correction fluid. Acute intoxication may lead to arrhythmia, hypoxia, electro-lyte imbalance, and death (so-called "sudden sniffing death"). *(Ref. 3, p. 900; Ref. 4, pp. 257–263)*

16. (d) A series of stages that people usually go through when try-ing to stop addictive behaviors was suggested by Prochaska and DiClemente. These stages are: precontemplation, contem-plation, preparation, action, and maintenance. Recognition of a higher power belongs to the 12-step program (Step 2). Motivational interviewing, a nonconfrontational counseling approach developed by Miller and Rollnick (1991), has been used as one treatment modality in patients with alcohol and substance use disorders. *(Ref. 3, pp. 903–904)*

17. (b) Bulimic patients have a higher risk for developing sub-stance and alcohol abuse than patients with anorexia, restrict-ing type. Adolescents with substance/alcohol abuse comorbid with other psychiatric disorders have higher risk for relapse. Posttraumatic stress disorder and depression are associated with alcohol dependence in female adolescent patients, who usually experience longer depressive episodes, demonstrat-ing more conduct problems, and psychosocial and academic impairments. Substance abuse, especially comorbid with mood disorders, conduct disorder, and personality disor-ders, increases suicide risk. Sexual abuse is also associated with more serious drug and alcohol involvement. *(Ref. 3, pp. 905–907)*

18. (e) After evaluating patients, the stages of drug involvement should be determined and different treatment levels of care (developed by the American Society of Addiction Medicine) provided to individual patients. Substance abuse treatment approaches are different for children and adolescents than for adults. Family involvement is crucial. Multisystemic therapy treating substance-abusing delinquents shows more favorable outcomes than probation or counseling. Compared to interac-tional groups, CBT groups show better short-term outcomes although they show no superiority at the 15-month follow-up. *(Ref. 1, pp. 800–805; Ref. 3, pp. 901–905)*

19. (b) Program focus, delivery technique, evaluation and train-ing, and support are essential aspects of effective interven-tions. Targeting different populations with different focuses using a variety of techniques, many prevention programs have been developed, used, and examined, with some more effec-tive than others. Programs with informational or affective components are *less* effective than those that use social influ-ence and life skills approaches. *(Ref. 3, pp. 908–909)*

20. (c) Research data regarding the pharmacological treatment of youth with dual diagnoses are limited. Studies show lithium is found to be efficacious in reducing alcohol use in adolescents with bipolar disorder and comorbid substance dependence. Fluoxetine is effective in treating depression in drug-depen-dent delinquents. Studies also show treatment of ADHD in adolescents decreases future risk of developing substance use disorders. Alternatives, such as Strattera, Wellbutrin, clonidine, and guanfacine can be tried for youth with ADHD comorbid with a substance use disorder. However, stimulants may be used with careful monitoring in this population if alternatives are unsuccessful. *(Ref. 3, pp. 907–909)*

10

SPECIAL ISSUES (SUICIDE, SEXUALITY, AIDS, ADJUSTMENT DISORDER, ABUSE, PERSONALITY DISORDERS, ELECTIVE MUTISM, AND STUTTERING)

QUESTIONS

Directions: Select the best response for each of the questions 1–55.

1. Which of the following statements regarding lethality of suicide among children and adolescents is *inaccurate*?

   a. Appraisal of the lethality of suicide intent is associated with the child's cognitive development.
   b. Perceived lethality by the child is associated with the level of the suicidal risk.
   c. Demographic characteristics and psychological factors are relevant in determining the lethality of suicide.
   d. High medical lethality of suicide attempts is associated with female gender.
   e. Lethality of impulsive suicide attempts is associated with availability of more lethal methods, such as accessibility of firearms.

2. Suicide completion rates are the *highest* in which one of the following groups?

   a. White females
   b. White males
   c. Black females
   d. Black males
   e. Asian females

3. Based on current research, all of the following are suggested for youth suicide-prevention programs *except:*

   a. Gun control and decreased availability of lethal weapons
   b. Program to avoid negative impacts on children whose first-degree relatives are involved with suicide
   c. Increased media coverage of youth suicide
   d. Programs targeted at high-risk groups
   e. Educational campaigns to increase recognition of serious symptoms of depression

4. According to the DSM-IV-TR, all of the following are necessary to make the diagnosis of adjustment disorder *except:*

   a. An identifiable stressor occurs within 3 months of the onset of symptoms.
   b. The reaction to the stressor can appear to be normal or expectable.
   c. The disturbance must resolve within 6 months unless there is a chronic stressor.
   d. There must be significant impairment in functioning.
   e. No other psychiatric disorder can be present.

5. In cases of physical or sexual abuse, the reporting requirement is:

   a. Confirmed abuse after clinical evaluation
   b. Suspected abuse after clinical evaluation
   c. Suspected abuse after parental notification
   d. Any case of suspected abuse
   e. Any case of confirmed abuse

6. All of the following statements about the epidemiology of abuse and neglect of children and adolescents are accurate *except:*

   a. There are no data to show the exact incidence of child abuse in the United States.
   b. Physical abuse is reported more frequently than neglect.
   c. Reports made by physicians are more likely to be substantiated than those from other groups reporting abuse.
   d. Utilizers of public health care are more likely to be reported than those using private health care.
   e. Reporting of abuse is greater for minorities and the poor.

7. According to a 1998 report by the U.S. Department of Health and Human Services, which of the following most closely approximates the percentage of maltreatment fatalities in 1996 that involved children younger than age 3?

   a. 5 to 15%
   b. 15 to 30%
   c. 30 to 45%
   d. 45 to 60%
   e. More than 75%

8. All of the following statements regarding the epidemiology of sexual abuse are accurate *except:*

   a. Sexual abuse is not rare, and is more prevalent than perceived.
   b. Based on retrospective studies, 10 to 34% of girls are sexually victimized before age 18.
   c. Most sexually abused children are abused by someone unfamiliar to them.
   d. Females are more likely to be abused than are males.
   e. Boys are least likely to report the abuse if the perpetrator is a female.

9. The risk factors for child sexual abuse include all of the following *except:*

   a. Female gender
   b. Being approximately age 10 for females and age 9 for males
   c. Affluent economic status
   d. Single parenthood
   e. Positive parental history of childhood sexual abuse

10. All of the following statements regarding the profiles of perpetrators of sexual abuse are correct *except:*

   a. Selection of victimized children is based primarily on their sexual attraction.
   b. The victims are considered as their narcissistic extensions.

c. Appearance and age of the victims may match their own characteristics when they were first abused.

d. They are often described as passive and inadequate in most aspects of their life.

e. They tend to put themselves into situations where children can be accessed.

11. Which one of the following components of the evaluation and intervention of sexually abused children is *most* controversial?

a. Evidence collection and acute evaluation by Emergency Room (ER) physicians

b. Introduction of anatomically correct dolls

c. Avoidance of additional emotional trauma

d. The safety of the child

e. Notification of the proper authorities

12. The *most* common way by which a child acquires AIDS is:

a. Being born to a mother infected with the human immuno-deficiency virus (HIV)

b. Receiving a blood transfusion

c. Homosexual activity with an HIV-infected person

d. Kissing an HIV-infected person

e. Heterosexual activity with an HIV-infected person

13. The *most* common presentation of AIDS in young children is:

a. Fever

b. Lymphadenopathy

c. Recurrent otitis media

d. Persistent oral candidiasis

e. Failure to thrive

14. Which of the following ethnic groups has the *highest* incidence of HIV infection?

a. Whites and Hispanics

b. Blacks and Hispanics

c. Blacks and Whites

d. Blacks and Asians

e. Whites and Asians

15. All of the following statements regarding the gender identity disorder of childhood (GIDC) are accurate *except*:

a. The onset is typically before 5 years of age.

b. Psychopathology is greater than in the normal population.

c. Biologic abnormalities in sexual differentiation are rarely causative.

d. Most of these children are confused about their gender identity.

e. Internalization of emotions is more common than externalization of emotions.

16. In girls, GIDC is distinguished from their being "tomboys" by all of the following *except*:

a. Boyish behavior

b. Unhappiness with female gender status

c. Aversion to culturally defined feminine clothing

d. Verbalized discomfort with their sexual anatomy

e. Acted-out discomfort with their sexual anatomy

17. The *most* common sexual orientation outcome of GIDC in boys is:

a. Homosexuality

b. Homosexual transsexualism

c. Bisexuality

d. Heterosexuality

e. Transvestism

18. By what age do young people have a sense of who they are in relationship to others—that is, a sense of identity or personality?

a. 1 to 3 Years

b. 3 to 6 Years

c. 6 to 12 Years

d. 12 to 16 Years

e. 16 to 20 Years

19. Which of the following conditions is *least* likely to be comorbid with borderline personality disorder (BPD) in children?

a. Attention-deficit hyperactivity disorder (ADHD)

b. Anxiety disorder

c. Obsessive–compulsive disorder (OCD)

d. Major depressive disorder (MDD)

e. Posttraumatic stress disorder (PTSD)

20. What is the *earliest* age at which a child who meets the criteria for antisocial personality disorder may be given this diagnosis according to the DSM-IV-TR?

a. Any age as long as the criteria are met

b. 12 Years of age

c. 15 Years of age

d. 18 Years of age

e. 21 Years of age

21. The percentage of young people who stutter and spontaneously improve by adolescence or adulthood is:

a. 5 to 15%

b. 15 to 30%

c. 30 to 50%

d. 50 to 80%

e. 80 to 95%

22. Based on recent studies of completed suicide among adolescents, all of the following factors have been found to be associated with completed suicide *except*:

a. Presence of alcohol or substance abuse

b. The accessibility of firearms in their homes

c. A history of inpatient psychiatric treatment

d. The usage of lithium in depressed patients with bipolar disorder

e. Male gender

23. All of the following statements regarding suicide attempts and suicide rates among young people are accurate *except:*

    a. Due to the lack of a national registry, reliable national data for suicide attempts are not available.

    b. The age-adjusted rate of suicide among 15- to 24-year-olds continues to increase.

    c. Suicide is now the third leading cause of death among 15- to 24-year-olds.

    d. The rates of suicide attempts and suicide are higher among psychiatric patients than in the general population.

    e. The age-adjusted rate of suicide among 5- to 14-year-olds decreased in 2000 compared to that in 1992.

24. Explanations for the increase in youth suicide based on cohort and period effect include all of the following *except:*

    a. Increased divorce in the general population

    b. Increased depression in youth and the general population

    c. Increased substance abuse by youth

    d. Decreased numbers of youth in the population

    e. Greater intensity of competition

25. All of the following findings reflecting recent studies of psychopathology among randomly selected youth age 9 to 17 are accurate *except:*

    a. Suicidal ideation only is reported by 5.2% of youth.

    b. Having made a suicide attempt is reported by 3.3% of youth.

    c. Attempters are less likely to be sexually active than those who only have suicidal ideation.

    d. Attempters experience more stressful life events.

    e. Having attempted suicide or suicidal ideation were both associated with the presence of psychiatric disorders.

26. Based on current research, all of the following statements regarding the biological etiology of suicidal behavior are correct *except:*

    a. A higher level of CSF 5-HIAA is found in suicidal people.

    b. There is lower whole blood tryptophan content among inpatient children with a recent suicide attempt.

    c. Adolescent suicide attempters have lower platelet benzodiazepine receptor densities.

    d. Suicidal inpatient children have higher levels of plasma cortisol during the dexamethasone suppression test.

    e. Depressed patients with history of suicide attempts secrete more growth hormone.

27. All of the following statements regarding risk factors for youth suicidal behavior are correct *except:*

    a. Suicide attempters have more lifetime and recent stressful events.

    b. Suicide victims are more likely to have family members with suicidal tendencies.

    c. Suicidal adolescents are more likely to have a positive family history of mood disorders, violence, and substance abuse.

    d. Physical abuse and sexual abuse are risk factors for suicide.

    e. Strong ethnic identification is associated with increasing suicide rates.

28. Conditions and disorders often associated with adolescent suicide include all of the following *except:*

    a. Developmental disorders with impaired learning skills

    b. Low intelligence

    c. Borderline personality disorder

    d. Antisocial personality disorder

    e. Narcissistic and schizoid traits

29. In considering stress reactions, all of the following mental disorders usually preclude the diagnosis of adjustment disorder *except:*

    a. Uncomplicated bereavement

    b. Personality disorders

    c. Psychological factors affecting physical condition

    d. PTSD

    e. OCD

30. All of the following statements regarding the outcome for children and adolescents with adjustment disorders are accurate *except:*

    a. Adolescents have poorer outcomes than do adults.

    b. Most adolescents (>70%) do well.

    c. Symptoms of adjustment disorder in youth are more likely to progress to other, more severe mental disorders.

    d. Outcome diagnosis cannot usually be predicted from the initial diagnosis.

    e. Disturbance of conduct predicts poorer outcome than disturbance of mood.

31. Which of the following is the *least* common characteristic of physical abuse?

    a. Burns

    b. Multiple injuries at similar stages of healing

    c. Ruptured viscera

    d. Head and eye injuries

    e. Rib fractures and spiral fractures

32. Which of the following characteristics is *least* commonly seen in physically abusing parents?

    a. Social isolation

    b. Environmental stress

    c. Violence between parents

    d. Suicidal ideation

    e. Use of alcohol and drugs

33. Which of the following psychiatric disorders and conditions is *least* commonly associated with childhood physical abuse?

    a. PTSD

    b. Attachment dysregulation

    c. Aggression

    d. Obsessive–compulsive disorder

    e. ADHD

34. Which of the following recommended treatments for physical abuse is *least* appropriate?

    a. Immediate removal of the child from the home

    b. Intervention in facilitating more secure attachment

    c. Family-based therapy

    d. Play therapy

    e. Group psychotherapy

35. All of the following statements regarding sexual abuse are accurate *except:*

    a. Sexual abuse is associated with low-income families.

    b. Victims tend to perceive their parents as rejecting, and not nurturing.

    c. Psychiatric disorders found among abused children include anxiety, depression, PTSD, aggression, and poor self-esteem.

    d. The majority of adults with dissociative identity disorder have a childhood history of abuse.

    e. Victims of sexual abuse are more inhibited in their sexual activities with fewer numbers of sexual partners.

36. Which of the following statements regarding sexual abuse of males is accurate?

    a. Boys are less likely to be abused by strangers than are girls.

    b. Sexual abuse is more likely to be reported by males than by females.

    c. Women are more likely to be the perpetrators.

    d. If the perpetrator is a male, the victimized boy may worry about being considered as homosexual.

    e. If being abused by a female, boys are more likely to be supported by caregivers.

37. According to Finkelhor and Browne (1986), the extent to which a child is traumatized by sexual abuse is related to a combination of all of the following factors *except:*

    a. Traumatic sexualization

    b. Powerlessness

    c. Suicidality

    d. Stigmatization

    e. Feelings of betrayal

38. Which of the following factors is found to be the *most* significant predictor of internalizing and externalizing behavioral problems in victims of sexual abuse?

    a. Poor mother–daughter relationship

    b. Concurrence of physical and sexual abuse

    c. Maternal psychiatric status

    d. The number of family-related stressors

    e. Age at the time of sexual abuse

39. Studies have found all of the following factors can mislead pre-schoolers who are suspected victims of sexual abuse during interviews *except:*

    a. If they feel they should "guess" or "pretend."

    b. If they feel their memories are "weak."

    c. If they do not fully understand the adults' language.

    d. If the interviewers are considered as friendly.

    e. If the interviewers have bias about the events.

40. Which of the following psychiatric diagnoses is most consistently reported with sexual abuse as compared with other mental disorders?

    a. MDD

    b. PTSD

    c. Somatization disorders

    d. Generalized anxiety disorder

    e. Substance abuse disorders

41. All of the following statements regarding physical abuse of children are accurate *except:*

    a. Definitions of physical abuse may be different across cultures.

    b. Abused children are more likely to be diagnosed with depression, conduct disorder, alcohol abuse, and attention-deficit disorders.

    c. Parents of abused children are more likely to have a psychiatric disorder.

    d. Abusive behaviors are more often found in fathers who have attempted suicide.

    e. Adolescents with histories of suicide attempt are more likely to be reported as victims of physical abuse.

42. Which of the following symptoms is *least* likely to be associated with sexually abused children?

    a. Venereal disease

    b. Compulsive masturbation

    c. Precocious sexual knowledge

    d. Prepubertal vaginal bleeding

    e. Late onset of menarche

43. Which of the following is *least* necessary to make the diagnosis of HIV/AIDS in children younger than 13 years?

    a. History of a risk factor associated with HIV/AIDS

    b. Presence of craniofacial dysmorphism

    c. Lymphoid interstitial pneumonia and pulmonary lymphoid hyperplasia

    d. Evidence of HIV infection

    e. Laboratory evidence of immunodeficiency

44. Which of the following statements regarding neurologic symptoms or evidence of encephalopathy related to HIV infection in children is *inaccurate*?

    a. The infection involves a failure to achieve new developmental milestones or loss of milestones.

    b. It involves cognitive impairment.

    c. It can present as being apathy with emotional lability.

    d. It is an uncommon occurrence in this population (<20%).

    e. It involves language impairment.

45. Adolescents who are at increased risk of acquiring HIV infection include all of the following *except:*

a. Those who have been sexually active with high-risk partners
b. Those who use illicit drugs, especially injecting drugs
c. Those who use condoms
d. Gay adolescents
e. The recipients of blood transfusion

46. All of the following statements regarding the pharmacological treatment of HIV infection are correct *except:*

a. All the antiretroviral drugs have potential side effects.
b. All the antiretroviral drugs are safe to combine with psychotropic medications due to lack of drug–drug interactions.
c. The antiretroviral drugs may cause abnormal lipid profiles.
d. The antiretroviral drugs may cause disturbance of glucose metabolism.
e. The antiretroviral drugs may cause redistribution of body fat.

47. All of the following statements regarding GIDC are accurate *except:*

a. The disorder is associated with a distinct hormonal abnormality.
b. Parents of GIDC boys are more likely to describe their sons as beautiful than are parents of control boys.
c. College students rate boys with GIDC significantly more attractive and rate girls with GIDC less attractive.
d. Parents of GIDC children are more tolerant of cross-gender behavior.
e. Fathers of boys with GIDC spend less time with their sons.

48. Which of the following therapies are proven *most* efficacious in the treatment of GIDC?

a. Individual psychotherapy
b. Family therapy
c. Cognitive therapy
d. Behavior therapy
e. None of the above

49. Which of the following findings is *least* likely to help make the diagnosis of borderline personality disorder in children?

a. Restricted development in relationships, affect, and cognitive functioning
b. Transient visual and auditory hallucinations
c. Severe separation anxiety and schizoid retreat and social withdrawal
d. Subjective distress regarding important life choices
e. Chronic regression state

50. Multimodal treatments of borderline personality disorder usually include all of the following *except:*

a. Individual therapy
b. Parental/family therapy
c. ECT
d. Pharmacological interventions

e. Partial and inpatient hospitalization, and residential programs

51. All of the following statements regarding selective mutism are accurate *except:*

a. The child refuses to speak in specific social situations.
b. The child does not usually speak at home.
c. Educational and interpersonal functioning is impaired.
d. The disorder typically starts between 3 and 8 years of age.
e. The female to male ratio is 2:1.

52. Selective mutism has been considered a symptom or a subtype of which of the following conditions in children?

a. ADHD
b. Social phobia
c. Schizophrenia
d. Personality disorder
e. Conduct disorder

53. The *least* necessary differential diagnosis to be considered in evaluating selective mutism is:

a. Pervasive developmental disorder
b. ADHD
c. Hearing impairment
d. Mental retardation
e. Developmental language disorder

54. Which of the following possible etiologies has received the *least* empirical support as a cause of stuttering?

a. Genetic
b. Neurologic
c. Behavioral
d. Family dynamics
e. Psychotropic medication

55. All of the following are phases originated from the Tasker's stage model of disclosure by parents of children with HIV/AIDS diagnoses *except:*

a. Ambivalence phase
b. Secrecy phase
c. Exploratory phase
d. Readiness phase
e. Disclosure phase

Matching

56–58. Choose one from the following phrases that describes the condition most accurately.

a. Pattern of erotic responsiveness
b. Sense of self as male or female
c. Adoption of male and female cultural markers

56. Gender identity
57. Gender role
58. Sexual orientation

ANSWERS AND EXPLANATIONS

1. **(d)** Females are relatively more likely to attempt suicide and males are usually reported as more likely to make a more medically lethal attempt or successful suicide attempt. It is important to evaluate the demographic characteristics and psychological factors that are relevant in determining the lethality of a suicide attempt. Lethality is also associated with male adolescents with affective or substance abuse disorder and the accessibility to lethal methods (in impulsive attempts). Due to cognitive immaturity, children may not fully appreciate the lethality of suicide methods. It is crucial to evaluate both objective and perceived lethality. Children may be at higher suicidal risk if the perceived lethality is higher than the objective lethality. *(Ref. 1, pp. 891–892; Ref. 3, pp. 796–797)*

2. **(b)** White males have the highest rate of suicide completion in the general population. Among adolescents and young adults ages 15 to 24, suicide is the third leading cause of death, and the sixth leading cause for children ages 5 to 14. *(Ref. 3, pp. 796–797)*

3. **(c)** Studies show that increased suicidal attempts in youth are associated with the recent media coverage (2 weeks after the event) of youth suicide. To minimize the contagion or imitation effect and prevent confusion and fear, organized liaison approaches with media and promotion of helpful media coverage of the event are recommended. *(Ref. 1, pp. 898–899; Ref. 3, p. 803)*

4. **(e)** Other psychiatric disorders may be present, but the disturbance under consideration should not meet the criteria for any other specific mental disorder. *(Ref. 4, pp. 679–683)*

5. **(d)** All states now have laws that require professionals to report all cases of suspected abuse immediately. While parents should be informed that abuse is suspected and that an investigation will take place, it is not required to do so before notifying the authorities. *(Ref. 2, pp. 217–218)*

6. **(b)** Neglect accounts for 53.5% of reports, physical abuse for 22.7%, and sexual abuse for 11.5%, with one fourth of total cases involved with more than one type of maltreatment. No data of the exact incidence of child abuse in the United States are available due to the reporting biases and investigatory procedural constraints. Abuse reports are more likely to be filed for ethnic minorities, poor and urban residents, and utilizers of public health care. Investigatory agencies are more likely to substantiate reports from physicians than from other groups reporting abuse. *(Ref. 3, p. 1209)*

7. **(e)** More than 75% of fatalities due to maltreatment in 1996 involved younger children (less than age 3), so it seems that younger children are at greater risk for fatal maltreatment. *(Ref. 1, p. 837)*

8. **(c)** Most abuse occurs with someone familiar to the child. Victims of sexual abuse are most likely to be abused by a male parent or male parent figures. The prevalence of sexual abuse is higher than commonly perceived and it is not rare, unfortunately. Retrospective studies show alarmingly high rates, with 10 to 34% of girls being victimized during their childhood. The gender ratio is approximately 4:1 with females at higher risk. When being victimized by female perpetrators, boys are less likely to report. *(Ref. 1, pp. 854–855; Ref. 3, p. 1217)*

9. **(c)** Lower economic status (not affluent status) is one of the child sexual abuse risk factors among others listed, including female gender, being approximately 10 years old in females and 9 years old in males, single parenthood, and parental history of childhood sexual abuse. *(Ref. 3, p. 1217)*

10. **(a)** Perpetrators tend to select their victims primarily based on their emotional needs more than sexual attraction, and they select victims that match the age and appearance of themselves when they were first abused. They view their victims as their narcissistic extensions; they are often described as passive and inadequate, although they are found to seek circumstances and events where children can be accessed. *(Ref. 3, pp. 855–856)*

11. **(b)** The use of anatomically correct dolls to provide definitive evidence is controversial. Most experts agree that they should not be introduced to the child in isolation as a diagnostic test, and should be used with caution. The most important aspect of evaluation and treatment is the safety of the child. Proper authorities should be called. The child should not be returned to the home unless the perpetrator is no longer there and/or the nonperpetrating parent or guardian can protect the child. ER physicians who are trained in conducting sexual abuse evaluation should do initial evaluation and evidence collection. Guidelines for the necessary physical examination after sexual abuse are outlined by the American Academy of Pediatrics (Shaw, 1999). *(Ref. 1, pp. 857–858; Ref. 2, pp. 219–220; Ref. 3, pp. 1219–1220)*

12. **(a)** Ninety-one percent of pediatric AIDS cases are the result of children being born to mothers who are intravenous drug abusers and/or the sexual partners of HIV-infected males, and 4% of all pediatric AIDS cases are the result of blood transfusions or receiving tissue donations. Kissing an HIV-infected person is not known to cause AIDS. Breastfeeding carries a risk of 7 to 22%. The recent reduction in the pediatric AIDS incidence and fatality rates is attributable to early recognition and treatment, and prevention of vertical transmission from mother to child. *(Ref. 1, pp. 873–874; Ref. 3, p. 1176)*

13. **(e)** Failure to thrive with loss of developmental milestones is the most common presentation of AIDS in young children. Other presenting symptoms include those listed, plus fever, recurrent bacterial infections, opportunistic infections, chronic unexplained diarrhea, hepatomeglia, spleenomeglia, and evidence of neuroencephalopathy. *(Ref. 1, p. 876)*

14. **(b)** Blacks and Hispanics are overrepresented among both pediatric and adolescent AIDS patients. The reduction of the incidence and fatality rates is low in African-American and Hispanic populations. Urban areas with >500,000 people

constitute 85% of all pediatric AIDS cases. *(Ref. 1, p. 873; Ref. 3, p. 1176)*

15. (d) Most children "know" that they are male or female with only some being confused about their gender identity. The psychopathology rate among GIDC is similar to that of psychiatric control children, but greater than in the normal population. *(Ref. 1, pp. 817–819; Ref. 2, pp. 155–156; Ref. 3, pp. 726–727)*

16. (a) Boyish behavior occurs both in tomboys and in girls with GIDC. However, girls with GIDC, as compared with tomboys, are unhappy with their female status, have an aversion to culturally defined feminine clothing, and verbalize or act out discomfort with their sexual anatomy. *(Ref. 1, p. 820; Ref. 3, pp. 730–731)*

17. (a) Follow-up more than 10 years after the diagnosis of GIDC in boys found that 75% were classified as homosexual (attracted to persons of the same biological sex) or bisexual. Homosexuality is the most common long-term outcome of GIDC in boys. *(Ref. 1, p. 830; Ref. 3, pp. 731–732)*

18. (c) While identity consolidation is a task of adolescence, children have a sense of themselves as independent beings with their own personal history and way of being by 6 to 12 years of age. *(Ref. 1, pp. 778–779)*

19. (c) Children with BPD may have other comorbid axis I diagnoses, such as ADHD, anxiety disorder, MDD, or PTSD. All of those listed and others, such as conduct disorder, somatization disorder, schizophrenia, and partial complex seizures, should be considered in the potential differential diagnosis while evaluating patients with BPD. *(Ref. 3, pp. 891–892)*

20. (d) Although the DSM-IV-TR states that there must be evidence of a conduct disorder before the age of 15, it specifies that the age at the diagnosis must be at least 18 years. Other personality disorders can be diagnosed prior to age 18 if they meet the criteria according to the DSM-IV-TR. *(Ref. 1, p. 789; Ref. 4, pp. 701–706)*

21. (d) Stuttering is usually a transient developmental phenomenon in early childhood and improves in 50–80% of all young people. *(Ref. 2, p. 206)*

22. (d) Lithium has been shown effective in reducing suicidal attempts in patients with depression and bipolar disorder. Discontinuation of lithium is associated with an increased risk of suicide. Due to the lethality of lithium overdose, its use in children and adolescents should be closely supervised and monitored by responsible adults. Accessibility of lethal weapons is associated with complete suicide, which may also explain the gender difference in complete suicides (females tend to use other ways, such as ingestion of drugs). History of psychiatric hospitalization and presence of alcohol or substance abuse are also associated with suicide. *(Ref. 1, pp. 894–896; Ref. 2, p. 216; Ref. 3, pp. 796–803)*

23. (b) The suicide rate among 15- to 24-year-olds has almost tripled since the 1950s; it peaked in 1977, and has been decreasing in the last few years. While national rates of suicide attempts are not available, national data on suicide still show an alarming fact that suicide is the third leading cause of death among 15- to 24-year-olds. The suicide rate among 5- to 14-year-olds decreased in 2000 compared to that in 1992, although it has been fluctuating a little in the last few years. The rates of suicide and attempts are both higher in psychiatric patients (especially those with a history of inpatient treatments) than in community samples, and there is an association between the lethality of attempts and the severity of symptoms of mood disorder. *(Ref. 1, pp. 894–895; Ref. 3, pp. 796–797)*

24. (d) An increase in the number of young people during certain historical periods (period effect) in the general population has been correlated with an increased suicide rate and is referred to as the cohort effect. An explanation is that the increased number of young people increases competition, and thus anxiety and stress. *(Ref. 1, p. 895; Ref. 3, pp. 796–797)*

25. (c) In a recent study of psychopathology in a randomly selected youth sample sponsored by NIMH, 3.3% reported having attempted suicide and 5.5% reported only suicidal ideations. Compared to the suicidal ideation reporters, the suicide attempters are more likely to become sexually active, smoke cigarettes and marijuana, and experience more stressful life events. However, both groups are associated with having psychiatric disorders, such as mood, anxiety, or disruptive disorders. *(Ref. 1, p. 896)*

26. (a) Many studies have shown that low levels of CSF 5-HIAA are associated with suicidal behaviors, indicating a possible etiological involvement of aberrant serotonin system functioning. All other statements listed are accurate, based on some recent studies attempting to elucidate the biological factors of suicidal behaviors. *(Ref. 3, p. 800)*

27. (e) Strong cultural affiliation (not ethnic identification) was found to predict the suicide attempts in a community study of Native Hawaiian adolescents. Recent or lifetime stressful events, family history of mood disorders, substance abuse, physical and sexual abuse, violence, and suicidal behaviors are all associated with suicidal behavior in youth. *(Ref. 3, pp. 800–801)*

28. (b) No research supports that low IQ is associated with increased suicidal behavior. Increased risk is associated with youth with developmental disorders having learning difficulties, personality disorders, and deficits with impulse control. *(Ref. 3, p. 799)*

29. (e) An individual with a nonstress-related axis I disorder, such as OCD, can develop into an adjustment disorder when he or she encounters a significant stress. For example, an individual can develop an adjustment disorder after parental divorce, which is comorbid with OCD. However, all of the other listed diagnoses generally exclude a diagnosis of adjustment disorder. The exception is if new symptoms develop as a result of a new stressor. Other diagnoses to be considered in evaluating possible adjustment disorder include those listed, plus conditions not attributable to a mental disorder that are a focus of attention or treatment, and specific disorders such as anxiety or mood disorders. *(Ref. 1, pp. 767–768; Ref. 2, p. 170; Ref. 4, pp. 681–682)*

30. **(b)** Over 70% of adults with a diagnosis of adjustment disorder are found to be well at follow-up as compared with 44% of adolescents. The adjustment disorder symptoms can last longer than 6 months if chronic stressors persist, and can progress to other, more severe mental disorders, such as major depressive disorder, which occurs more frequently in youth than in adults. The outcome diagnoses vary widely and cannot be predicted from the presenting symptoms of the initial diagnosis. However, some diagnostic subtypes such as disturbance of conduct can predict poorer outcomes. *(Ref. 1, pp. 769–770; Ref. 2, pp. 169–170; Ref. 4, p. 681)*

31. **(b)** Multiple injuries with various (not similar) stages of healing are more characteristic of physical abuse. Other characteristic injuries include bruises in the configuration of fingers or a belt, spiral fractures, subdural hematoma, radiographic evidence of old fractures, and multiple rib fractures. *(Ref. 1, pp. 840–841; Ref. 2, p. 219; Ref. 3, p. 1209)*

32. **(d)** Suicidal ideation is a frequent finding among abused children, but not among their parents, although mothers are reported to be depressed. Other characteristics include borderline or subaverage intelligence, unemployment, overcrowding, social isolation, psychiatric disorders, and violence between parents, alcohol/substance abuse, and inappropriate expectations of the child. *(Ref. 1, p. 839; Ref. 2, pp. 218–219; Ref. 3, p. 1210)*

33. **(d)** Obsessive–compulsive disorder is not commonly associated with physical abuse. Other characteristics of abused children include anxiety disorders and PTSD, cognitive and neurological impairments, dissociative disorders, ADHD, depression and suicide, self-destructive behavior, impaired impulse control and aggression, and impaired social relations. *(Ref. 1, pp. 843–846; Ref. 2, p. 220)*

34. **(a)** While removal of the child from the home has often been the case in the past, it is possible for many children to stay in the home (unless the child's safety is in jeopardy) when the abusing parent is engaged in treatment and there are frequent home visits. The treatment goals are first to protect the child and to strengthen the family. Interventions that can facilitate secure attachment between the child and parent are recommended. Other recommended approaches include appropriate educational placement, family-based therapy, psychotherapies (either in individual or group settings), and play therapy. Symbolic reenactments of the abuse often occur in play therapy, allowing for safe displacement of complex thoughts and emotional feelings so that the child can work through them, developing healthy coping strategies and eventually being healed. *(Ref. 1, pp. 847–848; Ref. 2, p. 220; Ref. 3, pp. 1213–1214)*

35. **(e)** Victims of sexual abuse have difficulty in modulating their sexual impulses, involving more risk-taking behaviors, and having greater numbers of sexual partners, earlier onset of sexual activity, and more frequent unprotected sex. Sexual abuse is associated with low income, limited parental education, and social disruption. The victims often view their parents as rejecting and not nurturing. As listed in the question, many psychiatric disorders and conditions correlate with sexual abuse. Dissociation may occur, which can inter-

fere with cognitive performance. Most adults with dissociative identity disorder have a history of childhood abuse. *(Ref. 3, pp. 1217–1218)*

36. **(d)** If being abused by males, the victimized boy may worry about being considered as homosexual. Studies also show victimized boys are more likely to identify as homosexual. Compared to girls, boys are more likely to be abused by strangers and not to have reported the abuse. Women are less likely to be the abusers; men are still more likely to be the perpetrators of sexual abuse against boys. If being abused by females, the victimized boys are less likely to report the abuse or be supported by caregivers when they do. *(Ref. 1, pp. 855–856)*

37. **(c)** Suicidality and other externalizing behaviors, along with a variety of emotional and behavioral symptoms, may occur in youth who are victims of sexual abuse. But suicidality is not one of the factors proposed by Finkelhor and Browne to describe the extent to which children are traumatized by sexual abuse. Premature stimulation can result in inappropriate, early sexual behavior (sexualization); powerlessness can lead to anxiety, fear, and feelings of helplessness; stigmatization may result from the discovery of the abuse or from the reactions of others; and a feeling of betrayal may result from being misused by someone who was trusted. *(Ref. 1, p. 856)*

38. **(a)** Hazzard et al. (1995) found the only significant predictor of internalizing and externalizing problems following abuse is a poor mother–daughter relationship. Other reports on child sexual abuse indicate certain conditions are associated with overall poorer outcomes, including: maternal psychiatric status predicting the outcome of sexually abused children, the number of family-related stressors predicting PTSD, the age at the time of abuse predicting an increased severity of emotional and behavioral symptoms, family adaptability and responses to the disclosure of abuse predicting intensity of the child victim's symptoms, and concurrence of physical and sexual abuse predicting an increased severity of sexualized behavioral problems. *(Ref. 3, p. 1218)*

39. **(d)** Studies have shown false memories of sexual abuse may occur, especially in preschoolers who are more vulnerable to be confused during faulty interviews. Along with other situations listed in the questions, when the interviewers are seen as unfriendly (not friendly), intimidating, or authoritarian children are more likely to be misled during the interviews. *(Ref. 3, p. 1220)*

40. **(b)** While a variety of mental disorders may occur in the victims of sexual abuse, PTSD is the most consistently reported compared to others. *(Ref. 3, p. 1218)*

41. **(d)** An association between suicide and abuse is identified and studies find that mothers with a history of suicide attempts are more likely to have child-abusive behaviors. According to different cultural practices and cultural values, physical abuse can be defined differently. The definition we use is based on Public Law 100-294. Victims of physical abuse are more likely to be diagnosed with depression, conduct disorder, and attention-deficit disorders, and are more likely to maltreat their offspring. Abusive parents are more likely to be diagnosed with a psychiatric disorder. *(Ref. 3, pp. 1208–1210)*

42. (e) Early onset of menarche has been reported in sexually abused girls. Other symptoms that should raise the suspicion of abuse include lacerations or other injuries to the anus or genitals, recurrent urinary-tract infections, pregnancy, running away, sleep disturbance, and somatic complaints. *(Ref. 1, pp. 857–858; Ref. 2, pp. 221–222; Ref. 3, p. 1219)*

43. (b) According to the Centers for Disease Control, the diagnosis is based on three essential factors to define HIV/AIDS in children younger than 13 years, including history of a risk factor, lab evidence of immunodeficiency, and evidence of HIV infection, with recurrent bacterial infections, lymphoid interstitial pneumonia, and pulmonary lymphoid hyperplasia being considered as indicative of AIDS infection. While there are a variety of central nervous system manifestations of AIDS in children and suggested embryopathy attributed to *in utero* HIV infection, craniofacial dysmorphism has not been confirmed. *(Ref. 1, p. 876; Ref. 3, p. 1177–1178)*

44. (d) Encephalopathy is consistently noted in approximately 65% of HIV-infected children. A series of complications of encephalopathy is found, such as loss of developmental milestones, failure to achieve normal neurological development, cognitive deteriorations, attention deficits, language impairments, and emotional lability. *(Ref. 1, p. 876; Ref. 3, pp. 1177–1178)*

45. (c) Using condoms and abstinence are protective factors that prevent developing an HIV infection. Adolescents who are sexually active with multiple partners and those who engage in unprotected sex are at greater risk. Male adolescents who have sex with males have higher risk, and using illicit drugs and injecting drugs are significant risk behaviors. Even though blood banks started screening for HIV, there are still some reported new AIDS cases in adolescents and adults who have received blood transfusions. *(Ref. 1, pp. 877–878; Ref. 3, p. 1177)*

46. (b) There are potential drug–drug interactions between psychotropic medications and antiretroviral agents. Potential side effects such as disturbance of lipid and glucose metabolisms and lipodystrophy syndrome should be monitored while treating patients with antiretroviral agents, and potential drug–drug interactions should be considered. *(Ref. 3, p. 1178)*

47. (a) No identifiable hormonal abnormality has been found in GIDC. While GIDC boys spend less time with both their fathers and mothers than do normal controls, they report feeling closer to their mothers. Boys with GIDC are more likely than non-GIDC boys to be described as beautiful. Based on pictures of children with GIDC, college students rate boys as more attractive and girls as less attractive compared to their same gender controls. *(Ref. 1, pp. 823–826; Ref. 3, pp. 727–728)*

48. (e) A number of interventions have been utilized in treating children with GIDC, including behavioral therapy, parental counseling, family and group therapy, and psychodynamic psychotherapy. Due to the lack of randomized, controlled clinical trials it is still unclear which one is the most efficacious approach. *(Ref. 1, pp. 828–829; Ref. 3, p. 731)*

49. (d) Subjective distress can occur in other mental disorders and does not usually help diagnose borderline personality disorder in children. Transient hallucinations are more common in borderline adolescents than in borderline adults. Children with borderline personality disorder may rapidly regress when encountering stress, which may lead to a loss of contact with reality; sudden suicidal ideation and behaviors; overwhelming, intense rage; and violent fantasies. Severe separation anxiety, schizoid retreat, and generalized restricted development may also present. *(Ref. 1, p. 782; Ref. 3, p. 891)*

50. (c) Many different interventions have been used for treating borderline disorder in children and adolescents without any available well-controlled studies indicating the best therapeutic modality. Due to the complex nature of the disorder, multimodal treatment approaches are proposed that rely on no single approach, but rather combine them when clinically indicated. ECT, however, has not been considered as one of the approaches. *(Ref. 3, pp. 892–893)*

51. (b) Children with selective mutism often speak at home. They selectively choose not to speak in specific social situations even though they are able to speak. Selective mutism is more prevalent in females than in males, and typically begins around 3 to 8 years of age. The symptoms usually resolve by age 10. *(Ref. 1, p. 596; Ref. 2, pp. 91–93)*

52. (b) Black and Uhde (1995) believe selective mutism is a symptom or a subtype of social phobia because of its presentation as fear of public speaking. *(Ref. 1, p. 596)*

53. (b) Children with ADHD usually do not present with selective mutism. Aphasia, schizophrenia, and conversion disorder also should be considered in the differential diagnosis. *(Ref. 1, pp. 596–597; Ref. 2, pp. 93–94; Ref. 3, pp. 616–617)*

54. (d) Stress related to family dynamics may exacerbate stuttering, but there is no evidence that indicates family dynamics cause stuttering. However, familial transmission is common and the risk of stuttering among first-degree relatives is three times higher than for the general population. Biological, neurological, behavioral, and psychotropic medication factors can all contribute to the etiology of stuttering. *(Ref. 2, p. 206; Ref. 3, p. 614)*

55. (a) The Yale Child Study Center Program for HIV Affected Children and Families enriched Tasker's five-stage model of disclosure with a developmental perspective identifying four phases that parents go through in disclosing the HIV/AIDS status of their children, including secrecy phase, exploratory phase, readiness phase, and disclose phase. Although AACAP recommends informing the infected children of HIV status, few protocols are available to guide the clinicians and family. Studies show disclosure has some beneficial effects on family functioning and may facilitate permanency planning. A recent study shows children who disclosed their HIV status to their peers have higher CD-4 cell counts, an indication of improved immune response. *(Ref. 3, pp. 1182–1183)*

56. (b) Gender identity is usually established by 3 years of age, and as early as 24 months. *(Ref. 1, p. 813)*

57. (c) Gender role is the adoption of male and female cultural markers, such as clothing, toy interests, fantasy play, mannerisms, and gender of playmates. It is typically established between 1 and 6 years of age, with girls having wider variability. *(Ref. 1, p. 813)*

58. (a) Sexual orientation may be heterosexual, homosexual, or bisexual. Most experts agree that it takes place after gender role and gender identity have been established, but the agreement is not universal. *(Ref. 1, p. 813)*

11

PSYCHOLOGICAL TESTING AND RATING SCALES

QUESTIONS

Directions: Select the best response for each of the questions 1–15.

1. All of the following statements regarding referral questions for psychological testing describe good practice *except:*
   a. Referral for assessment of a child's developmental process.
   b. Referral for assessment of a child's intellectual capacity and academic achievement.
   c. Referral for clarification of a child's diagnoses and assistance with therapeutic interventions.
   d. Referral questions should be explained to the parents.
   e. Referral questions should be formulated by the testing clinician after evaluation.

2. Which of the following is the *best* definition of construct validity on a testing instrument?
   a. The test's capacity to measure what it is supposed to measure
   b. The test's effectiveness in predicting an individual's performance in specific areas
   c. The fact that the test's content covers a representative sample for the property being measured
   d. The degree to which the test results can be reproduced
   e. Pretesting of the test on a large, demographically representative group of individuals

3. All of the following intelligence tests can be used reliably with children 4 years of age *except:*
   a. McCarthy Scales of Children's Abilities (MSCA)
   b. Kaufman Assessment Battery for Children (K-ABC)
   c. Stanford–Binet Intelligence Scale, Fourth Edition
   d. Wechsler Intelligence Scale of Children IV (WISC-IV)
   e. Peabody Picture Vocabulary Test–Revised (PPVT–R)

4. All of the following statements regarding the Vineland Adaptive Behavior Scale are accurate *except:*
   a. It is an excellent measurement of adaptive behavior.
   b. It assesses psychosocial functioning.
   c. It can be used with retarded individuals.
   d. It can be completed by the child's teacher.
   e. It measures academic achievement.

5. The Rorschach inkblots can be used for children as young as:
   a. 3 Years
   b. 6 Years
   c. 9 Years
   d. 12 Years
   e. 16 Years

6. Which of the following measures is *not* used for testing socio-emotional functioning for children and adolescents?
   a. Children's Apperception Test (CAT)
   b. Halstead–Reitan Neuropsychological Test
   c. Human figure drawing
   d. Sentence-completion tests
   e. Thematic Apperception Test (TAT)

7. All of the following instruments can be used during early infancy *except:*
   a. Bayley Scales of Infant Development
   b. Gesell's Developmental Schedules
   c. Denver Developmental Screening Test
   d. Brazelton Neonatal Behavioral Assessment Scale-2
   e. Machover Draw-A-Person Test (DAP)

8. Which of the following instruments has the *best* performance data and *greatest* usage in measuring childhood behavior problems?
   a. Missouri Assessment of Genetics Interview for Children (MAGIC)
   b. Child Behavior Checklist (CBCL) (Achenbach)
   c. Child Schedule for Affective Disorders and Schizophrenia (K-SADS)
   d. Diagnostic Interview Schedule for Children and Adolescents (DICA)
   e. Interview Schedule for Children and Adolescents (ISCA)

9. Neuropsychological evaluation is useful in the assessment of all of the following areas *except:*
   a. Overall cognitive functioning and language
   b. Motor function and visuomotor integrity
   c. Executive functions and perception
   d. Specific brain damage site
   e. Learning, memory, and academic abilities

10. All of the following areas can be reliably assessed in children and adolescents using psychological tests *except:*
    a. Intellectual ability
    b. Personality functioning
    c. Life expectancy
    d. Educational accomplishment
    e. Adaptive behaviors

11. Which of the following statements regarding intelligence tests is *inaccurate?*
    a. Intelligence tests measure both a global/overall capacity and separate/subscale abilities.
    b. Intelligence quotient testing is necessary for making a diagnosis of mental retardation.

c. The most widely used tests to assess intelligence and cognitive functioning are the Wechsler scales.

d. Individual IQ scores demonstrate wide variability after the age of 5 years.

e. IQ testing can be used to assist making diagnoses of specific learning disabilities.

12. Which of the following statements regarding the PPVT-R is *not* accurate?

   a. It assesses expressive language abilities.

   b. It is often used as a screening instrument to estimate verbal ability and intelligence.

   c. It relies on vocabulary skills as an indicator of overall intellectual capacity.

   d. It has excellent validity and reliability when used together with the Expressive Vocabulary Test (EVT).

   e. It is easy to administer, requiring 11 to 12 minutes to complete.

13. Which of the following tests is *not* a commonly used projective test for clinical hypothesis generation?

   a. Thematic apperception test

   b. Wisconsin card-sorting test

   c. Draw-a-person test

   d. Kinetic family drawing

   e. Sentence-completion test

14. All of the following statements regarding the difference between the Millon Adolescent Personality Inventory (MAPI) and the Minnesota Multiphasic Personality Inventory (MMPI) for use with adolescents are correct *except:*

   a. Administration time for the MAPI is shorter than for the MMPI.

   b. There are fewer questions in the MAPI than in the MMPI.

   c. The MAPI has two forms (MAPI-C and MAPI-G), and the MMPI has an adolescent version—MMPI-A.

   d. The MAPI has a longer history than the MMPI-A.

   e. The MMPI-A is standardized on normative populations that weigh toward less educated families.

15. Which of the following tests can be used to measure nonverbal intelligence?

   a. Kaufman Brief Intelligence Test (K-BIT)

   b. Stanford–Binet Intelligence Scale, Fourth Edition

   c. Leiter International Performance Scale, Revised (Leiter-R)

   d. PPVT-R

   e. EVT

Matching

16–20. Select from the following the description that best matches each psychological test or rating scale:

   a. Preschool intelligence test

   b. Modified Beck Inventory

   c. Neuropsychological screen

   d. Attention-deficit hyperactivity disorder (ADHD)

   e. Internalizers–externalizers

16. Bender Visual Motor Gestalt Test

17. Wechsler Preschool and Primary Scale of Intelligence, Revised (WPPSI-R)

18. Connor's Teacher Rating Scale

19. Child Behavior Checklist (CBCL)

20. Children's Depression Inventory (CDI)

ANSWERS AND EXPLANATIONS

1. (e) In order to ensure the efficiency and efficacy of the assessment, it is critical to develop a list of referral questions to be answered by the psychological evaluations. The specific relevant referral questions should be formulated by the referring clinician, and explained to the parents of the child being assessed. Several areas that referral questions commonly address are: assessments of developmental process, intellectual capacity, academic achievement, learning disabilities, diagnoses, treatments, and prediction of course of treatment. *(Ref. 3, pp. 555–556)*

2. (a) Answer **b** defines criterion-related validity, answer **c** defines content validity, answer **d** defines reliability, and answer **e** defines standardization. It is important to know the reliability and validity of a particular test in interpreting the results. *(Ref. 1, pp. 166–167; Ref. 3, pp. 557–558)*

3. (d) The WISC-IV (previous version WISC-III) is designed to be used for children 6 to 16 years of age. The MSCA is designed for children ages 2.6–8 years, the K-ABC for children ages 2.6 to 12.6 years, the Stanford–Binet for children ages 2 to adults age 23 years, and the PPVT for those ages 4 to adulthood. *(Ref. 1, p. 171; Ref. 2, pp. 16–17; Ref. 3, p. 558)*

4. (e) The Vineland does not measure academic achievement, as does the Woodcock–Johnson Psychoeducational Battery or the Wide Range Achievement Test. There is some reported fluctuation in means and standard deviations across age groups with the Vineland. *(Ref. 2, p. 18; Ref. 3, p. 564)*

5. (a) The Rorschach is used to assess personality organization and provides data regarding the child's developmental capacities for reality testing, integration of affect, and maturational level of object relations. It can be used to evaluate personality development in children as young as 3; it is not usually considered a valid measure of psychopathology until later. *(Ref. 3, pp. 559, 566)*

6. (b) In addition to Luria–Nebraska Neuropsychological Battery for Children (LNNB-C) and NEPSY Developmental Neuropsychological Assessment, Halstead–Reitan Neuropsychological Test Battery for Children is another measure of general neuropsychological functioning of children and adolescents. The rest of the tests listed are all measures of socioemotional functioning, and other such measures may include Roberts Apperception Test for Children and the Rorschach Inkblot Test. *(Ref. 1, pp. 173–174)*

7. (e) The Machover Draw-A-Person Test (DAP) can be used as a projective test in subjects 3 years old and up. The other tests listed are measures of neonate, infant, and toddler development, and can all be used during early infancy. *(Ref. 3, pp. 508, 519)*

8. (b) The CBCL has been considered a gold standard among behavioral rating scales. It is validated and is the most widely used instrument in research and clinical settings to measure a range of internalizing and externalizing behaviors. The K-SADS, MAGIC, ISCA, and DICA are diagnostic interviews, not behavior rating scales. *(Ref. 1, pp. 150–152; Ref. 3, pp. 545, 1400)*

9. (d) Variability in cerebral organization makes it impossible to determine that one specific brain region is involved or damaged, especially using one particular test. Neuropsychological testing is rarely used to find the "site of lesion" and brain regions are interrelated in a manner that makes it very unlikely that only one particular brain region is involved. All other areas listed are commonly assessed through neuropsychological testing. *(Ref. 1, pp. 171–172)*

10. (c) Psychological testing cannot assess life expectancy. All other listed areas can be reliably assessed by psychological testing. Psychological testing can also provide concrete, standardized data about language skills, visual–motor coordination, developmental level, neurocognitive functioning, and occupational interest and aptitude. *(Ref. 1, pp. 165–180; Ref. 3, pp. 555–571)*

11. (d) Individual IQ scores are relatively stable after about age 5, although there may be individual differences. The Wechsler scales are most widely used, and are derived from the Wechsler–Bellevue Intelligence Scale, of which the Wechsler Intelligence Scale for Children-IV (WISC-IV) is a downward extension. IQ testing is necessary for considering diagnoses of mental retardation, giftedness, and specific learning disabilities. *(Ref. 1, pp. 169–170; Ref. 3, pp. 560–563)*

12. (a) The Peabody Picture Vocabulary Test, Third Edition (PPVT-III), updated from the previous edition of PPVT, was published in 1959, and was later updated to PPVT-R in 1981. It has been used to measure receptive vocabulary. The Expressive Vocabulary Test (EVT) measures word retrieval and expressive vocabulary. Because of their short administration time and ease of use, both tests are often used for screening purposes in research and clinical settings. Used together, they achieve better validity and reliability. *(Ref. 2, p. 16; Ref. 3, p. 563)*

13. (b) The Wisconsin card-sorting test (not a projective test) is used to measure executive functioning and attention capacity. All of the other tests listed are projective tests useful for generating clinical hypotheses regarding children's feelings about themselves and their families. The information generated needs to be integrated into the clinical evaluation and cannot be used alone. *(Ref. 1, pp. 173, 177; Ref. 3, p. 559)*

14. (e) The MMPI-A, published in 1992, standardized on normative populations weighing toward better educated families in a high socioeconomic class. The MMPI-A takes 45 to 90 minutes to administer, has 478 items, and has unique clinical categories. Its adult version has been widely used since the 1940s. The MAPI, published in 1982, was specially designed for use with adolescents and standardized on relevant normative populations. The MAPI takes about 20 minutes to administer, has 150 items, and utilizes DSM-IV terminology. *(Ref. 3, pp. 567–568)*

15. **(c)** Among the tests listed, the Leiter International Performance Scale, Revised (Leiter-R) is the only one that can be used to measure nonverbal IQ. *(Ref. 3, p. 558)*

Matching

16. **(c)** The Bender Visual Motor Gestalt Test, like the Visual Motor Integration and Benton Visual Retention tests, measures visual–motor deficits and visual–figural retention. *(Ref. 3, p. 559)*

17. **(a)** The WPPSI-R is intended for use in children 3 to 7 years of age. *(Ref. 3, p. 558)*

18. **(d)** The Connor's Rating Scale is a measure of externalizing behaviors and is best known for use in the assessment of ADHD. *(Ref. 3, p. 635)*

19. **(e)** The CBCL uses factor-derived scores to classify behaviors as externalizing or internalizing. *(Ref. 1, p. 152)*

20. **(b)** The CDI is derived from the adult Beck Depression Inventory, written at first-grade level, being used for youth 7 to 17 years of age. *(Ref. 3, p. 1400)*

12

PSYCHOPHARMACOLOGY

QUESTIONS

Directions: Select the best response for each of the questions 1–46.

1. Which of the following factors is *least* likely to affect psychotropic drug disposition?
   a. Absorption
   b. Distribution
   c. Neurotransmission
   d. Metabolism
   e. Excretion

2. All of the following principles of medication management are applicable to treatment of children and adolescents *except:*
   a. Use only as a last resort.
   b. Intervention should be started early if indicated.
   c. Based on diagnosis, intervention should be focused on target symptoms.
   d. Patient and family should be informed about the risks, benefits, alternatives, and potential side effects.
   e. A drug should be started at the lower end of the therapeutic range.

3. Clomipramine (Anafranil) potentially benefits all of the following disorders *except:*
   a. Obsessive–compulsive disorder
   b. Attention-deficit hyperactivity disorder (ADHD)
   c. Trichotillomania
   d. Obsessive–compulsive disorder (OCD)-like symptoms in children with autism
   e. Self-injury and stereotypic behaviors

4. Based on our current knowledge, all of the following statements regarding using amphetamine and methylphenidate in the treatment of ADHD are correct *except:*
   a. Amphetamine is Food and Drug Administration (FDA) approved for children as young as 3 years of age.
   b. They both invariably worsen tics when used in children with ADHD comorbid with tic disorders.
   c. In general, an effective dose of amphetamine is lower than that of methylphenidate.
   d. Methylphenidate blocks the reuptake of dopamine and facilitates the release of stored dopamine.
   e. Amphetamine more specifically facilitates the release of newly synthesized dopamine in addition to blocking its reuptake.

5. All of the following statements regarding long-acting stimulants are true *except:*
   a. They do not cause insomnia.
   b. The peak levels come later than with immediate release formulations.

   c. Amphetamine agents are twofold more potent than methylphenidate agents.
   d. Usually children do not need to take a dose in school, which can enhance compliance.
   e. They may minimize the rebound phenomenon commonly seen in immediate release formulations.

6. Monoamine oxidase inhibitors (MAOIs) are sometimes useful in the treatment of all of the following disorders in adolescents *except:*
   a. Bulimia nervosa
   b. ADHD
   c. Atypical psychosis
   d. Atypical and refractory depression
   e. Depression with prominent anxiety features

7. All of the following are considered good management practices in the treatment of neuroleptic-induced dyskinesias *except:*
   a. Lowering the dosage for akathesia and rabbit syndrome
   b. Discontinuing or lowering the dosage for tardive dyskinesia (TD)
   c. Using antiparkinsonian agents for acute dystonic reactions
   d. Lowering the dosage for neuroleptic malignant syndrome
   e. Slowly titrating dosage to avoid extrapyramidal reactions

8. All of the following statements regarding using clonidine in treating ADHD are correct based on current knowledge *except:*
   a. It should not be stopped abruptly.
   b. Combining it with methylphenidate agents will cause sudden death.
   c. It may help children with comorbid tics.
   d. Rebound hypertension may occur.
   e. Rebound hyperactivity, irritability, and tachycardia may occur.

9. Relative contraindications to the use of the beta-blocking agent propranolol include all of the following *except:*
   a. Asthma
   b. Diabetes mellitus
   c. Bradycardia, cardiac conduction defects, and heart failure
   d. Hypothyroidism
   e. Seizure disorder

10. All of the following statements regarding using carbamazepine in the treatment of seizure and mood disorders of youth are correct *except:*
    a. The therapeutic drug level of carbamazepine is well established in treating bipolar disorder in youth.
    b. Carbamazepine may cause Stevens–Johnson syndrome.

c. Carbamazepine has significant drug–drug interaction potential.

d. Carbamazepine can cause teratogenic effects.

e. Carbamazepine should not be considered as a first-line mood stabilizer.

11. All of the following medications have proven effective and useful in the treatment of bulimia *except:*

a. Phenelzine

b. Desipramine

c. Fluoxetine

d. Buproprion

e. Imipramine

12. All of the following statements regarding the differences between typical and atypical antipsychotics reflect the current state of our knowledge *except:*

a. Atypical antipsychotics have mixed interactions with dopaminergic and serotonergic receptors.

b. Atypical antipsychotics are more effective for negative symptoms.

c. Typical antipsychotics are helpful in mood regulation due to their thymoleptic properties.

d. Typical antipsychotics are more likely to cause extrapyramidal symptoms.

e. Some atypical antipsychotics show efficacy in treatment of aggression in children with autism.

13. Which part of a routine medical workup is *least* necessary prior to lithium administration?

a. Creatinine

b. Blood urea nitrogen (BUN)

c. Thyroid studies

d. Electroencephalography (EEG)

e. Electrolytes

14. All of the following statements regarding atomoxetine (Strattera) reflect the current state of our knowledge *except:*

a. It has both noradrenergic reuptake inhibiting and dopaminergic properties.

b. The FDA approved it for treatment of ADHD in both children and adults.

c. It can increase diastolic blood pressure and heart rate.

d. It can have drug–drug interactions with MAOIs and cytochrome (CYP) 2D6 inhibitors.

e. No data show that it causes growth suppression.

15. All of the following statements regarding pharmacokinetics in youth are correct *except:*

a. Infants, children, and adolescents are heterogeneous in drug distributions.

b. Gonadal hormonal changes during puberty may change drug plasma levels.

c. To achieve comparable plasma drug levels, children require smaller weight-adjusted doses of most medications.

d. With less acidity in their stomach contents, children absorb acidic drugs more slowly and weakly.

e. The relative volume of extracellular water is higher in younger children than in older ones; lithium level can be lower in younger children.

16. Which of the following statements about drug interactions and the CYP P450 system is *incorrect?*

a. It is important to consider potential drug interactions when using polypharmacy.

b. The CYP system is classified based on the similarity of their amino acid sequencings.

c. Genetic factors influence CYP-based drug metabolisms.

d. Not all psychotropic drugs undergo both phase I and phase II reactions.

e. Some African Americans are "somewhat slow" metabolizers of 2D6.

17. All of the following statements regarding the differences in psychopharmacologic treatments between youth and adults are true *except:*

a. Adolescents are more likely to experience dystonic reactions to antipsychotics.

b. Selective serotonin reuptake inhibitors (SSRIs) may have higher activating effects on prepubertal children.

c. Despite unfavorable side effect profiles of tricyclic antidepressants (TCAs), youth respond to TCAs more effectively.

d. Development may affect how psychotropic medications work.

e. Drugs may have shorter half-lives in youth than in adults.

18. All of the following principles should guide prescribing psychotropic medications for youth *except:*

a. Be aware of the limitations of the current psychiatric categorical diagnostic classification.

b. Obtain data from multiple informants.

c. Use closed-ended questions to elicit side effects from medications.

d. Collaborate with patients' caregivers.

e. Use pharmacological treatments in context as part of a multimodal treatment plan.

19. The *least* likely reason for resistance to taking psychotropic medication and noncompliance by a young person and his or her family is:

a. The implication of being "weird" or "crazy"

b. Lack of a perceived need for the medication

c. Lack of understanding of the disorder

d. A single daily dose

e. Media influence

20. Which of the following ADHD medications carries an FDA black box warning for risk of hepatotoxicity?

a. Pemoline (Cylert)

b. Ritalin

c. Concerta
d. Adderall
e. Dexedrine

21. All of the following statements regarding drug rebound in children with ADHD who are being treated with stimulant medications are accurate *except:*

a. A return to baseline behavior beginning sometime after the last dose of a stimulant may be due to drug rebound.
b. Insomnia may be due to drug rebound.
c. Insomnia may reflect the action of a stimulant.
d. A late afternoon or evening dose of a stimulant may be useful for reducing rebound.
e. Avoiding a long-acting formulation may help reduce rebound.

22. The *least* likely side effect of a stimulant is:

a. Stomachaches
b. Irritability
c. Hypotension
d. Slowed growth
e. Insomnia

23. Which of the following presentations in a patient is *least* likely to cause a clinician to switch from a stimulant to nonstimulant medication in treating youth with ADHD?

a. Anxious and affective symptoms
b. Sleep disturbance on stimulants
c. Significant substance abuse risk
d. Tics
e. Conduct disorder (CD) as a comorbid condition

24. The *least* accepted indication for treatment with antidepressant medication monotherapy is:

a. Separation anxiety disorder
b. School phobia
c. Enuresis
d. Psychosis
e. OCD

25. Medical management for tricyclic antidepressants includes all of the following *except:*

a. A baseline ECG
b. A repeated ECG at dosages > 3.0 mg/kg/day
c. A blood drug level at steady state
d. Monitoring of creatinine
e. Tapering when discontinuing the drugs

26. The *least* likely side effect of tricyclic antidepressants (TCAs) includes which of the following:

a. Shortening of the PR interval
b. Tooth decay
c. Hypotension
d. Prolonged QRS complex
e. Excessive sweating

27. All of the following statements regarding using desipramine to treat ADHD in children are correct *except:*

a. There are reports of sudden death in children treated with desipramine.
b. Preexisting cardiac abnormalities have been reported in children who died of sudden death.
c. Daily doses of more than 3.5 mg/kg increase the risk of asymptomatic ECG changes.
d. The highly selective serotonergic property of desipramine is responsible for its anti-ADHD effects.
e. Desipramine may prolong cardiac conduct time.

28. Which of the following antipsychotics does *not* induce dystonia?

a. Risperidone
b. Clozapine
c. Ziprasidone
d. Olanzapine
e. Aripiprazole

29. All of the following medical workups and monitoring should be considered when prescribing atypical antipsychotics *except:*

a. Fasting glucose
b. Creatinine
c. Lipid profile
d. Liver enzymes
e. Weight and waist circumference

30. Neuroleptic-induced Extrapyramidal Symptoms (EPS) and other severe side effects may include all of the following *except:*

a. Acute dystonic reaction
b. Akathisia
c. Muscle flaccidity
d. Neuroleptic malignant syndrome (NMS)
e. Tardive dyskinesia

31. Lithium has shown benefits in treating all of the following conditions in youth *except:*

a. Self-injurious behaviors in children with developmental delay
b. Bipolar disorder, type I
c. Treatment-resistant aggression
d. Aggressive behaviors in mentally retarded youth
e. Bipolar disorder comorbid with substance abuse

32. All of the following are common side effects of lithium seen during treatment *except:*

a. Gastrointestinal symptoms and weight gain
b. Tremor
c. Hyperthyroidism
d. Polyuria and polydipsia
e. Acne

33. Clonidine is often found helpful in treating all of the following disorders *except:*

a. Impulsivity and aggression

b. Posttraumatic stress disorder (PTSD)

c. ADHD

d. Psychosis

e. Tourette's disorder

34. When clonidine is used in the treatment of ADHD, all of the following are commonly noted *except:*

a. Improved attention

b. Decreased impulsivity

c. Decreased hyperactivity

d. Reduced emotional outbursts

e. Decreased comorbid tics

35. All of the following statements regarding the administration of clonidine reflect the current guidelines *except:*

a. Dosage begins with 0.05 mg at bedtime and progresses up to 0.2 to 0.3 mg a day.

b. Administration in children may be by transdermal patch lasting 4 to 5 days.

c. Pulse and blood pressure monitoring are essential.

d. Maximal response usually occurs within the first week.

e. It should be discontinued by gradual tapering.

36. The medical workup that should be completed prior to clonidine administration includes which of the following:

a. Complete blood count (CBC)

b. Electrolytes

c. Thyroid studies

d. EEG

e. Blood pressure

37. Which of the following is *not* a side effect of clonidine treatment?

a. Sedation

b. Orthostatic hypotension

c. Rebound hypotension

d. Confusion

e. Dry mouth

38. Propranolol is found to be helpful in the treatment of all of the following disorders *except:*

a. Impulsive aggression

b. Agitation and hyperarousal state related to PTSD

c. Akathisia

d. Anxiety

e. Depression

39. Coadministration of propranolol and which of the following drugs may cause a decreased metabolism of propranolol and an increased risk of excessive beta-blocking effects:

a. Fluoxetine

b. Lithium

c. Depakote

d. Risperidone

e. Lamictal

40. The *least* likely side effect of carbamazepine treatment is:

a. Liver dysfunction

b. Bone marrow suppression

c. Taratogenicity to a developing fetus

d. Cardiac conduction defects

e. Skin rash

41. Which of the following anticonvulsant agents is *unique* in its metabolism compared to others listed?

a. Divalproex sodium (Depakote)

b. Carbamazepine (Tegretol)

c. Gabapentin (Neurontin)

d. Lamotrigine (Lamictal)

e. Topiramate (Topamax)

42. Which of the following is the *most* concerning severe side effect of lamotrigine?

a. Weight change

b. Skin rash

c. Sedation

d. Agitation

e. Headache

43. Which statement regarding prescribing antipsychotics to treat irritability associated with autistic disorder in children accurately reflects current knowledge and research?

a. Low-potency neuroleptics are often useful.

b. Olanzapine has been approved by the FDA.

c. Research data show risperidone is often efficacious.

d. Haloperidol is contraindicated.

e. Weight gain is not an issue in children with autism.

44. Which of the following medications is considered as the first-line pharmacological treatment for panic disorder?

a. Alprazolam

b. Clonazepam

c. Imipramine

d. Fluoxetine (Prozac)

e. MAOIs

45. Psychopharmacologic agents that have demonstrated some benefits in the treatment of PTSD in youth include all of the following *except:*

a. Tricyclic antidepressants

b. Clonidine

c. SSRIs

d. Neuroleptics

e. Gabapentin

46. Which of the following medications has shown superiority to placebo in the treatment of anorexia nervosa in short-term inpatient trials?

a. Naloxone

b. Cyproheptadine

c. Clomipramine

d. Pimozide

e. Lithium

Matching

47–50. For each of the following medications, select the relative neurotransmitter effect that provides the best description of its action. Use each effect profile only once.

a. Primarily noradrenergic
b. Serotonergic and noradrenergic
c. Primarily serotonergic
d. Dopaminergic and noradrenergic

47. Venlafaxine

48. Clomipramine

49. Atomoxetine

50. Bupropion

51–54. For each of the following neuroleptics, select the profile that best describes its side effects. Use each side effect profile only once.

a. Relatively high risk of extrapyramidal symptoms
b. Blood disorder and seizure
c. Relatively low risk of EPS
d. QTc prolongation

51. Quetiapine (Seroquel)

52. Ziprasidone (Geodon)

53. Risperidone (Risperdal)

54. Clozapine (Clozaril)

ANSWERS AND EXPLANATIONS

1. (c) The therapeutic actions of psychotropic drugs depend on neuronal circuitry, synaptic neurotransmission, and intracellular information processing. However, neurotransmission is not a main factor that affects the disposition of drugs. Absorption, distribution, metabolism, and excretion are the four factors affecting drug disposition. *(Ref. 3, pp. 940–943)*

2. (a) Psychopharmacological treatment is considered part of an overall treatment plan and should not be used only when other interventions have failed. Instead, often the pharmacological therapy should be started early to avoid occurrence of complications, chronicity, and functional incapacitation. Informed consent should be obtained before starting a drug, and the lowest initiation and effective dose should be used to reduce the chance of having potential side effects that need to be monitored closely during treatment. *(Ref. 1, pp. 931–932)*

3. (b) Clomipramine has its greatest effect on the serotonergic system, which is abnormal in obsessive–compulsive disorder and trichotillomania (compulsive hair pulling). It also shows beneficial effects on OCD-like symptoms and repetitive behaviors in children with autism. It has not been effective in the treatment of ADHD. However, desipramine (a stronger noradrenergic agent) shows efficacy in treating ADHD. *(Ref. 1, p. 936; Ref. 3, pp. 962–963)*

4. (b) Some studies show stimulants can worsen tics. However, studies also show children with ADHD comorbid with tic disorders may not necessarily experience tic exacerbation during treatment with stimulants. Potential risks and benefits need to be considered in these situations. Even though more research data support the efficacy of methylphenidate agents in treating ADHD in children younger than 6, only amphetamine agents (such as Dexedrine and Adderall XR) have been approved by the FDA for use in children ages 3 and up. Although the exact mechanisms of stimulants are not fully understood, amphetamine agents seem to have a different mechanism of action than that of methylphenidate agents. *(Ref. 1, pp. 932–935; Ref. 3, pp. 958–960)*

5. (a) Long-acting preparation stimulant agents can still cause insomnia depending on the length of duration of different preparations, the time of administration, and metabolism of the drugs. In general, long-acting preparations are considered as effective as immediate-release agents, needing no additional dose during school time and minimizing noncompliance and behavioral rebound. *(Ref. 3, p. 959)*

6. (c) Atypical psychosis is not an indication for MAOIs. Strict adherence to a tyramine-free diet is necessary, and may be a problem for adolescents or for potentially suicidal or self-injurious patients. *(Ref. 1, pp. 936, 939, 965; Ref. 2, pp. 117, 281; Ref. 3, p. 966)*

7. (d) Discontinuation is necessary when symptoms of neuroleptic malignant syndrome are first present. The other neuroleptic-induced dyskinesias can be managed by lowering the dosage discontinuation, switching to alternative agents or using antiparkinsonian agents. *(Ref. 1, pp. 942–943; Ref. 2, pp. 302–304; Ref. 3, p. 962)*

8. (b) Review of data has not confirmed an association between sudden death and a combination of methylphenidate and clonidine. But the controversy continues, and caution is advised when using the combination. When stopping clonidine, it should be tapered over a period of several days to weeks to avoid rebound hyperactivity, irritability, hypertension, and tachycardia. *(Ref. 1, pp. 947–949; Ref. 2, p. 313; Ref. 3, p. 969)*

9. (e) Beta-blocking agents do not increase the likelihood of seizures. In fact, studies show the benefits of adding propranolol to anticonvulsant agents in children with seizure disorder and uncontrollable aggression. They do, however, affect all the other listed conditions that are considered as relative contraindications. *(Ref. 1, p. 949; Ref. 2, p. 314; Ref. 3, pp. 759, 956)*

10. (a) Carbamazepine was developed for its anticonvulsant effect, and no therapeutic level has been established for mood disorders. Young people with electroencephalogram abnormalities associated with behavioral indicators of organic personality disorder such as impulsivity, inattention, irritability, and aggressive behavior are sometimes helped by carbamazepine treatment. However, due to its side effect profile, drug–drug interaction potential, and lack of controlled studies to support its efficacy, carbamazepine should not be used as a first-line mood stabilizer. *(Ref. 1, p. 945; Ref. 2, p. 308; Ref. 3, p. 968)*

11. (d) Buproprion can decrease the seizure threshold and it should be avoided in bulimic patients. Imipramine, fluoxetine, desipramine, and phenelzine have all proven effective in the treatment of bulimia symptoms in weight-normal patients, even in those without depression. SSRIs are more advantageous than TCAs and MAOIs due to their overall better side effect profiles. *(Ref. 1, pp. 700–701; Ref. 2, p. 117; Ref. 3, pp. 697, 966)*

12. (c) Atypical antipsychotics are both dopaminergic (D2) and serotonergic (5-HT) and have thymoleptic properties, beneficial for mood disorder symptoms. While typical antipsychotics are mostly targeting positive symptoms, atypical antipsychotics are effective for negative symptoms as well. Atypical antipsychotics are less likely to cause EPS than typical antipsychotics. Most recently, the FDA approved risperidone for treating irritability associated with autistic disorder in children. *(Ref. 1, pp. 940–943; Ref. 3, pp. 960–962)*

13. (d) An EEG is usually not required prior to the administration of lithium. However, since preexisting cardiac conduction problems can be exacerbated by lithium, many recommend a baseline EKG. Repeat thyroid studies should be done every 6 months. A repeat BUN and creatinine should be obtained when polyuria, polydipsia, or persistent thirst appears. *(Ref. 1, pp. 943–944; Ref. 2, pp. 292–293; Ref. 3, p. 967)*

14. (a) Atomoxetine is mostly a noradrenergic reuptake inhibitor without dopaminergic property, and it is not a controlled substance. It may cause mild appetite suppression, but no data indicate long-term growth suppression. Having a better side effect profile compared to TCAs, it can still cause increased blood pressure and heart rate. Potential drug–drug interactions should be considered. *(Ref. 1, pp. 949–950; Ref. 2, p. 277)*

15. **(c)** Having an increased rate of metabolism and elimination, to achieve comparable drug levels, children usually need larger weight-adjusted doses of most medications. Absorption relies on pH-dependent diffusion and, having a less acidic stomach content, children absorb acidic medications more slowly and weakly. Total body water decreases with development, and younger children tend to have lower plasma concentrations of medications such as lithium. *(Ref. 3, pp. 939–941)*

16. **(e)** Among Caucasians, 7 to 10% have deficit CYP 2D6 causing less efficient metabolism of a number of psychotropic drugs. Some Asians (not African Americans) carry a genetic variant in 2D6 leading them to be "somewhat slow" metabolizers of 2D6. Some (2 to 3%) African Americans and Caucasians and 13 to 18% of Japanese are slow metabolizers of 2C19. *(Ref. 3, pp. 941–943)*

17. **(c)** Developmentally less mature noradrenergic pathways may be responsible for the lack of efficacy of TCAs in youth with depression. Selective serotonin reuptake inhibitors tend to be more activating in younger children, and adolescents are more likely than adults to experience dystonic reactions to antipsychotics. Metabolism and elimination are more rapid in young people, leading to shorter half-lives. The increased hepatic metabolic activity affects neuroleptics, while the increased renal clearance affects lithium. Children have a greater density of D_1 and D_2 receptors, which affects neuroleptic and tricyclic actions. *(Ref. 3, p. 951)*

18. **(c)** To elicit data on potential side effects of drugs, a combination of open-ended inquiry and inquiry on specific side effects should be used. Due to limitations of the current diagnostic classification system, children are often more heterogeneous in the etiologies and presentations of their psychopathologies, having a higher level of comorbidity. Multiple informants should be used to gather data and formulate assessment and a treatment plan, focusing on target symptoms. Engagement and collaboration of caregivers are essential for monitoring drug responses and side effects, and compliance enhancement. A combination of pharmacological therapies with other interventions results in a more therapeutic multimodal treatment. *(Ref. 3, pp. 957–958)*

19. **(d)** The more complicated a schedule of drug administration is, the less compliant patients become. Patients and their families may become more resistant or noncompliant when they think that taking medications implies being sick ("crazy" or "weird") and when they do not understand the disorders the medications are treating and the need for the treatment. Media influence can also confuse public perception and worsen compliance. *(Ref. 2, p. 263; Ref. 3, p. 957)*

20. **(a)** Hepatotoxicity occurs in 1 to 3% of patients treated with Cylert, which is why the FDA black box warning requires monitoring of liver enzymes. Cylert is only considered as a third-line drug in treating ADHD. *(Ref. 1, p. 934; Ref. 2, p. 275; Ref. 3, p. 660)*

21. **(e)** Using a long-acting agent, adding a smaller dose in the afternoon, and adding clonidine or guanfacine may be useful for reducing rebound. Insomnia may be due to rebound, or it may reflect the action of the stimulants. *(Ref. 1, p. 935; Ref. 2, p. 275; Ref. 3, pp. 660–661)*

22. **(c)** Stimulants can cause potential hypertension and tachycardia. Other side effects may include decreased appetite, stomachaches, sleep disturbance, slowed growth, palpitations, weight loss, headaches, irritability, and dysphoria. *(Ref. 1, pp. 932–935; Ref. 2, pp. 273–274; Ref. 3, pp. 660–661)*

23. **(e)** Youth with ADHD comorbid with CD usually respond to stimulants. Instead of switching off stimulants, more often they may need additional agents to target other underlying psychopathologies, such as anxiety, affective symptoms, psychosis, agitation, and aggression. Nonstimulants, such as TCAs, atomoxetine, buproprion, clonidine, and guanfacine, among others, can be considered as alternatives to stimulants in these situations. *(Ref. 1, pp. 950–957; Ref. 3, p. 661)*

24. **(d)** Monotherapy using antidepressants to treat psychosis even in a major mood disorder with psychotic features is not advised. Occasionally, serotonergic agents may worsen psychosis. Antidepressant monotherapy can be considered in the other conditions listed. *(Ref. 1, pp. 935–940; Ref. 2, pp. 277–291)*

25. **(d)** Monitoring of creatinine, a measure of renal clearance, is not necessary for treatment with tricyclic antidepressants as they are cleared primarily by the liver. A baseline ECG should be repeated at dosages above 3.0 mg/kg/day or in the event of any change in cardiovascular status. Blood levels should be determined when the dosage is above 3.0 mg/kg/day (1.5 mg/kg/day for nortriptyline), or at maintenance dose, or when side effects raise a concern that the blood level may be high on a lower dosage. *(Ref. 1, p. 938; Ref. 2, p. 280; Ref. 3, p. 963)*

26. **(a)** Prolongation of the PR and prolongation of QRS complex and QTc intervals are potential cardiovascular effects of TCAs. Other side effects of tricyclic antidepressants may include anticholinergic effects; hypotension and, rarely, hypertension; tachycardia; and decreased seizure threshold. Dry mouth secondary to anticholinergic effects may promote tooth decay. *(Ref. 1, pp. 935–938; Ref. 2, pp. 278–280; Ref. 3, pp. 952, 962–963)*

27. **(d)** Just like atomoxetine, desipramine is a highly selective norepinephrine reuptake inhibitor, which makes it unique (compared to other antidepressants) in effectively treating ADHD symptoms. Reports of deaths of children being treated with desipramine, while not conclusive, suggest that preexisting abnormalities were present in the children, highlighting the need for a baseline ECG and judicious monitoring. Due to its side effect profile, desipramine is not considered a first-line treatment for ADHD. *(Ref. 1, p. 938; Ref. 2, pp. 278–280; Ref. 3, pp. 962–963)*

28. **(b)** Clozapine does not induce dystonia, with low risks of EPS and TD. Quetiapine has low risk of EPS. The other listed antipsychotics can all induce dystonia and other EPS even though

the incidence is lower compared to typical antipsychotics. *(Ref. 1, p. 941; Ref. 2, pp. 295–305; Ref. 3, p. 954)*

29. **(b)** Atypical antipsychotics are not metabolized through the kidneys, and it is not necessary to check creatinine in general. However, they are cleared through the liver; therefore, liver function studies are necessary. A few authorities also recommend a baseline ECG. Due to potential side effects (such as weight gain, diabetes, dyslipidemia, and metabolic syndrome), weight, waist circumference, lipid profile, and fasting glucose should be monitored. *(Ref. 1, pp. 942–943; Ref. 2, pp. 299–300; Ref. 3, pp. 961–962)*

30. **(c)** Muscle rigidity (not muscle flaccidity) is a common sign of EPS and is one of the serious side effects of antipsychotics among the other listed symptoms. Regular use of the Abnormal Involuntary Movement Scale (AIMS) is helpful in monitoring many of these side effects. NMS can be life threatening, and TD can be irreversible after discontinuation of the offending agent. *(Ref. 1, pp. 942–943; Ref. 2, pp. 302–304; Ref. 3, p. 962)*

31. **(a)** Data have not supported the efficacy of using lithium to treat self-injurious behaviors in children with developmental delay. Lithium has been used most frequently in the treatment of bipolar disorders (acute mania, mixed episodes, prophylaxis, and bipolar depression), bipolar disorder comorbid with substance abuse disorder, and aggression. However, youth with prepubertal onset bipolar disorder respond less favorably to lithium than do those with adolescent onset. *(Ref. 1, pp. 943–945; Ref. 2, pp. 291–292; Ref. 3, pp. 966–967)*

32. **(c)** Goiter or hypothyroidism (not hyperthyroidism) may occur. Other common side effects of lithium treatment include diarrhea, gastrointestinal symptoms, polyuria, polydipsia, tremor, sleepiness, headaches, possible renal damage, acne, and weight gain. *(Ref. 1, p. 943; Ref. 2, pp. 294–295; Ref. 3, p. 967)*

33. **(d)** Clonidine is an alpha-adrenergic stimulating agent that inhibits noradrenergic activity. While it has been found useful in a number of disorders (including the other listed conditions), it is not generally helpful in the treatment of psychosis. In addition to the other disorders listed, it is also helpful in the treatment of other tic disorders, oppositional behaviors, and self-injurious behavior. *(Ref. 1, pp. 947–949; Ref. 2, pp. 311–312; Ref. 3, pp. 969–970)*

34. **(a)** Clonidine does not generally help attention problems in treatment of ADHD. Clonidine is noted to reduce emotional outbursts, impulsivity, and hyperactivity. Clonidine reduces the tics in patients with ADHD comorbid with Tourette's disorder or other tic disorders. *(Ref. 1, p. 956; Ref. 2, pp. 311–312; Ref. 3, p. 969)*

35. **(d)** Response may be delayed 2 to 4 weeks, and maximum benefits may occur a few months after initiation of the drug. If no effects are noted, the maximum tolerable dose should be given for 2 to 8 weeks before it is discontinued. Pulse and blood pressure should be monitored and tapering is needed if the drug is discontinued. *(Ref. 2, pp. 312–313)*

36. **(e)** A physical examination (including orthostatic blood pressure and heart rate) is necessary along with a review of systems and history of cardiovascular disease. An ECG is advised in very young children, if there is reason to suspect cardiovascular disease, and when clonidine and Ritalin are combined. Contraindications to clonidine use are history of syncope, bradycardia, and heart block. *(Ref. 2, pp. 312–313)*

37. **(c)** Rebound hypertension (not hypotension) and rebound hyperactivity can occur. The most common side effect is sedation. Other side effects may include dysphoria, depression, confusion, dry mouth, rash, abdominal pain, decreased glucose tolerance, and local irritation with a patch. *(Ref. 1, p. 948; Ref. 2, p. 313; Ref. 3, p. 969)*

38. **(e)** Propranolol has not been found helpful in treating depression. However, it is a nonselective beta-adrenergic receptor blocking agent that has been helpful in the treatment of aggressive behavior, uncontrollable rage and impulsive aggression, aggression secondary to organic brain syndrome and anxiety, and anxiety related to PTSD or phobia. It is also helpful in the treatment of akathisia. *(Ref. 1, pp. 948–949; Ref. 2, pp. 221, 313–314; Ref. 3, pp. 831, 956, 1220)*

39. **(a)** Coadministration of a beta-blocking agent (such as propranolol) with SSRIs can increase the blood level of the beta-blocker and its beta-blocking effect. *(Ref. 1, p. 949)*

40. **(d)** There is no indication that carbamazepine causes cardiac conduction defects. It is important that the medical workup and follow-up include evaluation of the liver and blood and rule out pregnancy. Skin rash, rarely, and Stevens–Johnson syndrome can occur. *(Ref. 1, pp. 944–945; Ref. 2, pp. 308–309; Ref. 3, p. 968)*

41. **(c)** Except for Neurontin, the listed anticonvulsant agents are metabolized through the liver and often are accompanied by more potential drug–drug interactions. Neurontin is excreted by the kidneys mostly unchanged, without significant drug interaction. Unfortunately, its efficacy as a mood stabilizer in youth has not been established. *(Ref. 3, pp. 968–969)*

42. **(b)** Skin rash can proceed to a full-blown Stevens–Johnson syndrome, which is a life-threatening condition. In children, Lamictal should be used extremely cautiously with very slow titration. *(Ref. 1, pp. 945–946; Ref. 3, pp. 968–969)*

43. **(c)** The FDA recently approved risperidone (not olanzapine) to treat irritability associated with autistic disorder in children. In this population, low-potency neuroleptics cause too much sedation and are less useful. Haloperidol, a high-potency neuroleptic, is very effective as well and is not contraindicated. *(Ref. 1, pp. 291–292, 963; Ref. 2, p. 196; Ref. 3, pp. 960–961)*

44. **(d)** Adult studies have reported the effectiveness of tricyclic antidepressants, MAOIs, and benzodiazepines in the treatment of panic disorder. Small-scale studies and reports of the treatment of panic disorder in children suggest that these agents are also of benefit for young people with the disorder. However, considering the side effect profile and safety issues, SSRIs are considered as the first-line agents in treating anxiety disorders in youth. *(Ref. 1, pp. 958–960)*

45. **(e)** There are no data to support the efficacy of gabapentin in treating PTSD. The other options listed have shown some benefits in treating PTSD in youth. In adults, the FDA has approved two SSRIs (paroxetine and sertraline) for treatment

of PTSD. In youth, SSRIs are considered as first-line agents even though no medications have yet been approved by the FDA for treatment of PTSD in youth. *(Ref. 1, pp. 628–631)*

46. (b) Cyproheptadine and amitriptyline have been found helpful in weight gain in inpatient trials. Clomipramine, lithium, thiothixene, pimozide, and naloxone have produced negative or equivocal results. *(Ref. 1, pp. 683–684)*

Matching

47. (b); 48. (c); 49. (a); 50. (d) In addition to the antidepressants listed: desipramine (primarily noradrenergic), and Trazodone and Nefazdone (both serotonin reuptake blockers and 5HT2A antagonists). *(Ref. 1, p. 949; Ref. 3, pp. 952–953, 963)*

51. (c) Seroquel has a relatively lower risk of EPS. *(Ref. 1, p. 941)*

52. (d) QTc prolongation has been associated with Geodon based on premarketing data. An EKG may be needed. *(Ref. 1, p. 942)*

53. (a) Among six atypical antipsychotics, risperidone is more like a high-potency typical agent, with a relatively high risk for EPS. *(Ref. 2, p. 303)*

54. (b) The prominent side effects of clozapine, used for treatment-refractory psychosis, include lowered seizure threshold, as well as granulocytopenia and agranulocytosis. *(Ref. 1, p. 941; Ref. 3, p. 954)*

13

PSYCHOTHERAPIES

QUESTIONS

Directions: Select the best response for each of the questions 1–26.

1. Melanie Klein's technique of child psychoanalysis is based on all of the following principles *except:*

   a. It is based on an unconscious fantasy life.
   b. Play is the child's mode of free association.
   c. Children can form a transference neurosis.
   d. Interpretation is central.
   e. Reassurance is used to lessen anxiety.

2. All of the following are characteristics of behavior modification treatment techniques *except:*

   a. Behaviors can be altered by new learning.
   b. Treatments focus on current behavior.
   c. There is a biopsychosocial focus.
   d. Treatment is directive and active.
   e. Assessment and evaluation are central characteristics.

3. Examples of specific disorders where behavior modification treatments have proven effective include all of the following *except:*

   a. Antisocial behaviors
   b. Encopresis
   c. Attention-deficit hyperactivity disorder (ADHD)
   d. Schizotypal disorder
   e. Phobias

4. Behavior modification has two general conceptual views, described as meditational and nonmeditational. All of the following statements describe the meditational view *except:*

   a. It focuses on direct connections between situational events and behavior.
   b. It emphasizes affects and cognition, which underlie behavior.
   c. Goals, beliefs, and self-statements play a critical role.
   d. It includes cognitive–behavioral approaches.
   e. It is not based solely on direct responses to environmental stimuli.

5. Favorable outcomes with focused time-limited psychotherapy are found in all of the following circumstances *except:*

   a. There is the ability to define a clear treatment focus.
   b. It enhances the patient's motivation and limits his or her nonadaptive dependency.
   c. It is especially good for children who have had serious losses and/or deprivation.
   d. The limited time frame is acknowledged.
   e. Both the patient and the therapist are engaged actively in treatment.

6. All of the following statements are useful and valid in developing a therapy group *except:*

   a. Poor social skills are a strong indication.
   b. Developmental level is a significant factor.
   c. Contraindications include extremely fragile children.
   d. Support groups work best with a mixture of disorders among the patients.
   e. Group therapy is usually possible with younger children.

7. Based on current research data, which of the following interventions is more effective than the others in treating depression in adolescents?

   a. Multifamily play group
   b. 12-Step group
   c. Cognitive–behavioral therapy (CBT) group
   d. Psychoanalytic group
   e. Psychodrama

8. All of the following individual psychotherapy approaches are likely to be helpful for children and adolescents with schizophrenia *except:*

   a. Developing healthy coping skills and defense mechanisms
   b. Strengthening reality testing
   c. Strengthening identity and adaptive behaviors
   d. Uncovering unconscious fantasies
   e. Providing education about the illness

9. All of the following are indications of countertransference that is interfering with a therapist's work with patients *except:*

   a. Failure to recognize the patient's developmental level, setting up unrealistic goals
   b. Recognizing a patient's transference feelings toward the therapist
   c. Ambivalent feelings about the patient secondary to the remnants of the therapist's own childhood relations with his or her past significant others
   d. Overidentification with the patient or parents resulting in rescue fantasies
   e. Permission for and encouragement of a patient's acting out

10. Which of the following psychotherapeutic treatments has the *least* evidence to support its effectiveness in the treatment of core symptoms of obsessive–compulsive disorder (OCD) in children and adolescents?

    a. Family therapy
    b. Psychodynamic psychotherapy
    c. Response prevention
    d. Systematic desensitization
    e. Cognitive–behavioral therapy

11. The *most* effective treatment for childhood-specific phobias is:

    a. Psychodynamic psychotherapy

    b. Beta-blockers

    c. Graduated exposure combined with contingency and self-control

    d. Benzodiazepines

    e. Family therapy

12. Anna Freud's system of psychoanalytic treatment varied from Melanie Klein's system in all of the following ways *except:*

    a. Play is not a substitute for free association.

    b. Children cannot form a true transference neurosis.

    c. Verbalization, educational efforts, and reassurance are utilized.

    d. Transference and resistance are interpreted.

    e. The key is to create a new relationship and promote normal development.

13. Psychodynamic psychotherapy with children and adolescents differs from psychoanalysis in all of the following ways *except:*

    a. The extent of support and guidance

    b. The activity of the therapist

    c. The relationship to the therapist

    d. The purpose of play

    e. It is a "watered-down" or lesser form of treatment

14. Criteria for termination of psychodynamic psychotherapy for children usually include all of the following *except:*

    a. The child has developed age-appropriate interests.

    b. The child achieves the expected academic level.

    c. The child is in a nonpathogenic environment.

    d. The child is progressing along a normal developmental path.

    e. The child is relatively symptom free.

15. All of the following treatment approaches have some empirical support for their efficacy or effectiveness in the treatment of conduct disorder *except:*

    a. Social skills training

    b. Problem-solving skills training

    c. Parent management training

    d. Psychodynamic psychotherapy

    e. Multisystemic therapy

16. Which of the following is the *best* researched and *most* promising treatment choice for youth with conduct disorder?

    a. Psychodynamic psychotherapy

    b. Parent management training

    c. Insight-oriented individual psychotherapy

    d. Group therapy

    e. Social skills training

17. Which of the following circumstances is the *least* appropriate indication for family therapy alone?

    a. More than one family member is symptomatic.

    b. One or more family members are at risk of decompensation.

    c. The identified patient is not motivated to participate.

    d. The dysfunctional interactions within the family contribute to presenting symptoms.

    e. The progress of individual therapy is stalled due to family system issues.

18. Parent management training has *less* positive outcomes in all of the following circumstances *except:*

    a. Low socioeconomic status

    b. Parental psychopathology

    c. Enmeshed social support network

    d. Marital conflicts

    e. Harsh punishments

19. All of the following guidelines regarding individual and group therapy that can be used with mentally retarded young people are correct *except:*

    a. Patients have to be verbal to benefit from the therapies.

    b. Therapies should be directive, concrete, and structured.

    c. An eclectic approach is needed.

    d. Individual or group therapies should be part of a comprehensive treatment plan.

    e. Realistic goals should be identified.

20. All of the following statements regarding behavior therapy programs for autistic individuals are correct *except:*

    a. Special attention must be given to generalization of behavioral changes.

    b. Long-term residential treatment is often needed for successful treatment.

    c. The therapy should be tailored individually.

    d. Promotion of social development is one of the goals.

    e. Early intensive intervention is crucial.

21. All of the following cognitive distortions in reasoning are associated with depression *except:*

    a. Arbitrary inference

    b. Selective abstraction

    c. Personalization

    d. Absolutistic thinking

    e. Responding to incorrect processing of information about the situation

22. Which of the following psychotherapy strategies used in children with separation anxiety disorder is *least* appropriate?

    a. Flooding

    b. Contingency management

    c. Cognitive strategies

    d. Modeling

    e. Family treatment

23. Which of the following reinforcements is *most* stable and resistant to change?

a. Continuous reinforcement
b. Intermittent reinforcement with a fixed interval
c. Intermittent reinforcement with a variable interval
d. Intermittent reinforcement with a fixed ratio
e. Immediate reinforcement

24. Psychotherapeutic techniques useful in the treatment of post-traumatic stress disorder (PTSD) include all of the following *except:*

a. Systemic desensitization
b. Avoiding traumatic reminders
c. Reworking guilt
d. Encouraging the interpretation of emotional reactions
e. Strengthening coping skills

25. The psychological treatment for anorexia nervosa *least* likely to be beneficial is:

a. Behavior therapy
b. Cognitive therapy
c. Supportive/psychoeducational therapy
d. Insight-oriented psychotherapy
e. Psychoanalytic psychotherapy

26. All of the following statements about group therapy for anorexia nervosa are accurate *except:*

a. Due to social avoidance, anorexic patients may show little interest in group therapy.
b. It is helpful for patients to learn that there are other people who have similar issues.
c. Outside contact among members is prohibited.
d. Chat rooms and group discussions on the Internet should be monitored.
e. Due to competition, significant weight loss may occur among group members.

Matching

27–30. Match the treatment name with the best treatment description. Use each description only once.

a. Emphasizing the establishment of boundaries within the family
b. Forcing confrontation of family conflicts among the family members to reach resolution
c. Focusing on the "unconscious" life of the family members
d. Identification of family rules, maintaining the family homeostasis, and strengthening the parental alliance

27. Triadic-based family therapy
28. Psychodynamic family therapy
29. Strategic family therapy
30. Structural family therapy

ANSWERS AND EXPLANATIONS

1. **(e)** Klein believed that play is a suitable substitute for the free association of adults and that children could form a transference neurosis despite their dependent and interactive relationship with their actual parents. She insisted that the analyst should provide only interpretations, without reassurance or guidance. *(Ref. 1, pp. 975–976)*

2. **(c)** The characteristics of behavior modification include its focus on overt behavior, learning, directive and active treatments, current determinants of behavior, assessment and evaluation, and the use of people in the everyday environment as treaters. Because of this specific focus, behavior modification is less likely to focus on broader issues included in a biopsychosocial context, although there may be indirect effects on this broader environment. *(Ref. 1, pp. 987–990)*

3. **(d)** According to the proponents of behavior modification, the technique can be used to treat any symptom that a child may experience. The disorder being treated must be defined in terms of one or two principal symptoms to be effectively measured and evaluated. To date, there have been no behavior modification programs specifically directed toward schizotypal disorder. *(Ref. 3, pp. 1005–1008)*

4. **(a)** The nonmeditational view focuses on direct (i.e., nonmeditated) connections between environmental or situational events and behavior. Operational conditioning represents a nonmeditational view. *(Ref. 1, pp. 985–986)*

5. **(c)** Time-limited therapy is relatively contraindicated in children and families where there is chronic severe pathology and where there are losses and deprivations. These conditions may be aggravated by focused, time-limited psychotherapy. Time-limited therapy can use different models based on various theoretical foundations. *(Ref. 2, pp. 327–328)*

6. **(d)** The composition of the group depends on the focus. Patients in support groups derive the most benefit if they share a stressor such as sexual abuse or focus on a particular psychiatric disorder such as conduct disorder. Mixtures of disorders among the patients work best in social skill groups. The developmental level is usually an important consideration in group assignment. *(Ref. 1, pp. 1033–1035; Ref. 2, pp. 335–337; Ref. 3, pp. 1024–1026)*

7. **(c)** Among the listed interventions, research supports the effectiveness of the CBT group over other approaches. *(Ref. 1, p. 1036; Ref. 3, p. 1030)*

8. **(d)** Therapeutic techniques are usually aimed at repressing primary process thinking rather than focusing on it. The therapist's roles include serving as an auxiliary ego and facilitating the child's understanding and appropriate expression of sensory perceptions. *(Ref. 1, pp. 399–400; Ref. 2, pp. 127–128; Ref. 3, pp. 751–752)*

9. **(b)** Misreading a patient's relationship to the therapist and misunderstanding of the patient's transference toward the therapist can interfere in therapeutic work with the patient. *(Ref. 3, p. 989)*

10. **(b)** While psychodynamic psychotherapy has not been shown to be effective in removing obsessions or compulsions, it can play an important role in addressing the way in which OCD has an impact on the person's life. Family therapy is important for both support and education and to improve family functioning, which improves the long-term outcome. A behavioral treatment such as response prevention, thought stopping, or desensitization is considered one of the treatments of choice, in addition to the use of selective serotonin reuptake inhibitors (SSRIs). *(Ref. 1, pp. 580–583; Ref. 3, pp. 841–843)*

11. **(c)** Childhood-specific phobias traditionally have been treated with psychodynamic psychotherapy, but graduated exposure combined with contingency and self-control approaches has proven the most effective. Psychopharmacologic treatment has not proven effective. *(Ref. 3, p. 825)*

12. **(d)** Freud did not accept play as a substitute for free association, as Klein did, nor did she believe that a true transference neurosis, where past relationships are relived through the analyst, happens in the same way with children as with adults. Efforts to decrease anxiety were acceptable to Freud. The interpretation of transference and resistance was central to both Freud's and Klein's techniques. *(Ref. 1, pp. 976–977)*

13. **(e)** Psychodynamic psychotherapy cannot be considered as a watered-down or lesser form of treatment compared to psychoanalysis, from which it was derived. Children in psychodynamic psychotherapy are given active support and guidance by a more active and available therapist. Play is not utilized primarily as a substitute for free association, but as a way for the child to communicate and form a relationship with the therapist, which may become the basis of a corrective emotional experience. *(Ref. 1, pp. 977–980)*

14. **(b)** Academic achievement is not considered one of the criteria for termination. Termination usually takes place after the child is making progress on his or her normal developmental path, living in a nonpathogenic environment, and has developed age-appropriate coping strategies, interests, interpersonal relationships, and behaviors. *(Ref. 1, p. 980; Ref. 3, p. 990)*

15. **(d)** Psychodynamic psychotherapy is not usually effective for treating conduct-disordered youth as they rarely acknowledge conflicts about their behavior. In social skills training, specific behaviors are developed to enhance the child's ability to influence his or her environment, obtain appropriate outcomes, and respond appropriately to the demands of others. Problem-solving skills training is focused on the child's perceptions, self-statements, attributions, and problem-solving skills. In parent management training, parents are trained to interact differently with their children. *(Ref. 1, pp. 518–519; Ref. 3, pp. 677–678)*

16. **(b)** Parent management training has proven to be the most effective and promising intervention in the treatment of youth with conduct disorder. Social skills training can be helpful. Psychodynamic psychotherapy and insight-oriented individual psychotherapy are not useful. Group therapy should be done with caution because antisocial behaviors can be contagious among youth. *(Ref. 1, p. 519; Ref. 2, pp. 52–53)*

17. **(b)** Family treatment can be useful in combination with other treatments when a family member is at risk of decompensation. Often, family therapy is part of a multimodal treatment plan, but there are circumstances when it can be used alone. Good indications for family therapy include when symptoms are present in more than one family member, psychological symptoms in one family member worsen when those in another improve with treatment, there is lack of motivation by the identified patient to change or engage in treatment, and individual treatment is blocked or retarded by family issues. *(Ref. 1, pp. 1015–1027; Ref. 2, pp. 332–333)*

18. **(c)** A limited or complete lack of social support network, among other circumstances listed, has been associated with less favorable outcomes of parent management training. In these circumstances, parents should focus on their own individual and marital problems while receiving maximally potent interventions. *(Ref. 1, pp. 1017–1018; Ref. 2, p. 331)*

19. **(a)** The patients do not have to be verbal to be eligible for individual or group therapies as long as they can somehow communicate with others. Individual psychotherapy might include supportive therapy, role modeling, and, to a lesser extent, psychodynamic principles. An eclectic approach is required and therapies are more directive, concrete, and structured, targeting more realistic goals, and being part of a comprehensive treatment plan. *(Ref. 1, pp. 252–253; Ref. 2, pp. 187–189; Ref. 3, pp. 608–609)*

20. **(b)** Because social development is one of the goals of treatment, a home-based approach is preferable to a residential placement. Since autistic children are handicapped in generalizing from one situation to another, attention must be given to both the school and the home. Behavior therapy programs need to be individualized since autistic children vary greatly in their handicaps and family circumstances. Research shows a long-term benefit from early intensive behavioral therapy, and it is critical to carry out such interventions across settings. *(Ref. 1, pp. 288–289; Ref. 3, pp. 593–594)*

21. **(e)** Responding to or acting on the incorrect processing of information about the situation is associated with anxiety disorder, such as in a phobia. All the other listed cognitive distortions are associated with depression. *(Ref. 3, pp. 1015–1016)*

22. **(a)** Flooding is rarely used in separation anxiety disorder. Gradual exposure and desensitization using relaxation are more appropriate approaches. All the other strategies listed can be used appropriately in treating separation anxiety disorder and recent research shows that CBT programs are particularly effective. *(Ref. 3, p. 824)*

23. **(c)** Intermittent reinforcements with a variable ratio or a variable interval are most stable and resistant to change. The intermittent reinforcements with a fixed ratio or interval are relatively less resistant to change. Continuous reinforcement provides rewards immediately after the occurrence of every single desired response, which is least likely to be stable and more vulnerable to change. *(Ref. 3, p. 1000)*

24. **(b)** Early psychotherapeutic work includes identifying feelings, reactions, and traumatic reminders. The recognition of the emotional meaning of the traumatic event is central to psychotherapeutic treatment. At times, systematic desensitization is needed. *(Ref. 1, pp. 626–627; Ref. 2, pp. 148–149)*

25. **(e)** Psychoanalytic psychotherapy by itself is largely ineffective in the treatment of eating disorders, especially because patients may view the silence of the traditional psychoanalysis as rejection. All the other listed interventions have been shown to be moderately effective in treating anorexia nervosa. *(Ref. 1, pp. 681–682; Ref. 2, pp. 109–111)*

26. **(c)** Through outside contact, members' self-worth and hope are reinforced, so members are encouraged to contact others outside the group. Group treatments have a higher dropout rate than does individual therapy. It is recommended that eating-disorder patients at widely different levels of development not be in the same group. Decreasing isolation and encouraging the sharing of thoughts and feelings are the main goals of group therapy. *(Ref. 1, pp. 682–683)*

Matching

27. **(b)** Triadic-based family therapy uses different strategies to force the conflicts into the open through confrontation among family members in order to reach a resolution. *(Ref. 1, p. 1012)*

28. **(c)** Psychodynamic family therapy focuses on the "unconscious" life of the family members and encourages them to share the unconscious conflicts and defenses, and intrafamilial transference reactions in the therapy. Psychodynamic family psychotherapy is good for families with long-standing but subtle symptoms, and it can be combined with individual therapies. Object relations theory is applied in psychodynamic therapy. To enhance the therapeutic process, attachment theory can be used as well to differentiate between "defensive" and "attachment" affects. *(Ref. 1, pp. 1012–1013)*

29. **(d)** Strategic family therapy sees families in terms of process and maladaptive problem-solving efforts. In the therapy, strategies should be developed to identify the family rules, strengthen parental alliance, and maintain the family's homeostasis. Paradoxical intervention, circular questioning, extended family intervention, and narrative therapy techniques can be used. *(Ref. 1, p. 1012; Ref. 3, pp. 1045–1046)*

30. **(a)** Structural family therapy focuses on adaptive and maladaptive structure, particularly in relation to power, boundaries, and preferred transactional patterns. Reestablishing and realigning boundaries is emphasized in the therapy. *(Ref. 1, p. 1011; Ref. 3, p. 1045)*

14

TREATMENT SETTINGS, HEALTH-CARE SYSTEM, AND OUTCOME

QUESTIONS

Directions: Select the best response for each of the questions 1–20.

1. The length of stay in the majority of inpatient psychiatric units is determined mainly by:
   a. Patient diagnosis
   b. Family stability
   c. Availability of less restrictive resources
   d. Funding availability
   e. Severity of illness

2. The *most* likely explanations for the recent trend reversing the increased use of inpatient care include all of the following *except:*
   a. The need for multiple integrated services
   b. Disproportionately high costs spent in inpatient services
   c. Publicity of a series of criminal and unethical scandals
   d. Focusing on intensive noninstitutional treatments
   e. Stricter statutory rights of minors

3. Milieu therapy is *best* described by which of the following?
   a. A French treatment based on the works of Lacan
   b. A special education program
   c. Utilization of the child's "life space" in treatment
   d. A form of environmental amelioration
   e. An eclectic, middle-of-the-road approach to treatment

4. All of the following are traditional groupings of length of psychiatric hospital stay *except:*
   a. Emergency: less than or equal to 3 days
   b. Acute: less than 2 weeks
   c. Short term: 1 to 3 months
   d. Intermediate: 3 to 5 months
   e. Long term: more than 9 months

5. All of the following dimensions in treatment programs are the factors accounting for the variability in outcomes among inpatient units *except:*
   a. Minimum square foot of space per patient
   b. Level of restrictiveness
   c. Length of stay
   d. Developmental level of patient
   e. Philosophy of treatment

6. All of the following are main components of treatment in a psychiatric hospital *except:*
   a. Individual therapy
   b. Pharmacotherapy
   c. Milieu therapy
   d. Psychoanalytic psychotherapy
   e. Family therapy

7. Common diagnoses for children receiving residential treatment include all of the following *except:*
   a. Adjustment disorders
   b. Depressive disorders
   c. Specific developmental disorders
   d. Pervasive developmental disorder, not otherwise specified
   e. Conduct disorder

8. The *most* significant factor associated with a successful outcome of residential treatment is:
   a. Family and community support
   b. Length of stay
   c. Amount of change during residential treatment
   d. Psychiatric diagnosis
   e. Planned discharge

9. Which of the following disorders in young children demonstrates the *greatest* improvement from outpatient individual behavioral psychotherapy?
   a. Obsessive–compulsive disorder
   b. Depression
   c. Phobias
   d. Conduct disorder
   e. Attention-deficit hyperactivity disorder (ADHD)

10. Which of the following is the *least* appropriate indication/criterion for inpatient psychiatric hospitalization of children or adolescents?
    a. Immediate physical danger to self
    b. Immediate danger to others
    c. Parent and child relationship problems and conflicts
    d. Failure of less intensive forms of treatment
    e. More intensive, systematic, and thorough evaluation that cannot be done in less restrictive settings

11. The *most* likely explanations for the large increase in proprietary psychiatric hospitals since the 1990s include all of the following *except:*
    a. Diminished availability of juvenile justice and child welfare
    b. Increased funding by private insurance and Medicaid
    c. Increased social instability
    d. Lesser scrutiny by third-party payers
    e. Looser statutory rights of minors

12. Jellinek and Herzog (1991) suggested a framework for guiding our pediatrician colleagues in helping parents of children with psychosomatic disorders to accept psychiatric consultation referrals. All of the following were suggestions they proposed *except:*

a. Wait to share a final etiologic diagnosis until all information is collected.
b. Suggest the interview is to gather further psychosocial information.
c. Do not refer resistant families.
d. Initiate a psychiatric consultation soon after hospitalization.
e. Suggest appropriate referrals to social service agencies if needed.

13. All of the following are guidelines for the child psychiatric emergency evaluation *except:*

    a. When in doubt, believe the caregivers' information over the child's.
    b. Obtaining information regarding both the child's current and baseline functioning.
    c. Performing a mental status examination.
    d. Determining the potential risk involved (danger to self or others).
    e. Developing a differential diagnosis, identifying interventions, and formulating a treatment and disposition plan.

14. Which of the following is considered to fall within the definition of partial hospitalization?

    a. Day care
    b. A therapeutic school
    c. A 24-hour-a-day hospital
    d. Day treatment program
    e. Group home

15. Common goals of day treatment include all of the following *except:*

    a. Alternative to hospitalization
    b. A step down from the hospital
    c. Intensive outpatient treatment
    d. Extensive evaluation
    e. Protection from acute suicidal intent

16. All of the following are principles that govern the discharge and aftercare planning for youth treated in partial hospital programs *except:*

    a. The least restrictive environment should be provided.
    b. Longer treatment is usually needed to reach optimal benefit.
    c. Maximizing a smooth and successful transition to new settings is needed.

d. Attention should be paid to termination.
e. Liaison with community resources and encouragement of compliance with follow-up is important.

17. All of the following statements regarding the effectiveness and outcome of partial hospitalization programs are accurate *except:*

    a. Day treatment is comparably as effective as residential treatment if there is a somewhat stable living arrangement.
    b. Gains in relationships and academic performance are noticed.
    c. Some 66 to 90% of children return to their home community.
    d. Older children show greater benefits than do younger ones.
    e. Family separation and out-of-home placement are associated with poor outcome.

18. Group homes are distinguished from residential treatment centers by all of the following *except:*

    a. They are larger in size.
    b. They rely more on community resources such as school.
    c. They provide less risk of institutionalization.
    d. They are more like a group living facility than an institution.
    e. There are fewer staff members per patient.

19. All of the following are common duties of child psychiatrists working in residential treatment programs *except:*

    a. Direct case consultation with the treating clinicians
    b. Complete responsibility for the treatment of the patients
    c. Participation in case conferences
    d. Direct psychiatric evaluation, medication management, and monitoring
    e. Medication rounds with facility nursing staff

20. All of the following are necessary protocols and procedures for psychopharmacologic therapy for youth in residential treatment programs *except:*

    a. Medical charts and records
    b. Written protocols for treatment with psychotropic medications
    c. Protocols for home visitations
    d. Protocols for lab studies and measurements
    e. Procedures for discharging patients on medications

ANSWERS AND EXPLANATIONS

1. (d) All of the possibilities listed affect the length of stay, but, unfortunately, recent studies have shown that funding availability or explicit program limitations are the major determinants of length of stay. *(Ref. 3, p. 1092)*

2. (e) The statutory rights of minors have been relaxed since the *Parham* decision making it easier for parents to hospitalize their children, which resulted in the increase of inpatient psychiatric admissions of children and adolescents in the mid-1970s. All the other situations listed account for the recent trend of reversing the increased use of inpatient care for youth. *(Ref. 3, pp. 1091–1092)*

3. (c) Milieu therapy is a treatment philosophy aimed at every aspect of the child's physical and social "life space" to create a multimodal therapeutic life experience. Early writers on the concept include Aichorn, Bettelheim, Redl, Wineman, and Trieschman. *(Ref. 2, p. 342; Ref. 3, p. 1094)*

4. (b) Length of hospital stay depends on the treatment programs and staffing of a hospital and the determinants of constraints on these dimensions. According to the traditional groupings of length of stay, less than 4 weeks is indicated for the acute condition. *(Ref. 3, p. 1092)*

5. (a) Minimum square foot per patient is a standard set by regulatory guidelines and is consistent across inpatient units. All of the other listed treatment dimensions in the question account for the variability in outcomes in inpatient units. Another dimension is hospital organization or affiliation. *(Ref. 3, p. 1092)*

6. (d) Individual, group, family, and milieu therapy, education, and pharmacotherapy are usually considered general components of psychiatric inpatient care. Special approval may be needed for others such as biofeedback and hypnotherapy. Due to the shortening of hospital stays, individual psychoanalytic psychotherapy (usually requiring a longer duration of treatment) is not a main component of treatment in most inpatient settings. *(Ref. 2, pp. 341–343)*

7. (a) Except for adjustment disorders, all of the diagnostic categories listed (in addition to ADHD and anxiety disorders) are commonly seen in residential treatment centers. Many of the children are wards of the state and have been abused or neglected. Delinquency and antisocial and aggressive behavior are often diagnosed as conduct disorder, which is a common indication for residential treatment. *(Ref. 3, p. 1097)*

8. (a) While all of the factors listed may be important in predicting outcome, by far the most significant factor is the extent of family and community support during enrollment, as well as the availability of help from community agencies and school programs. *(Ref. 3, p. 1102)*

9. (c) Disorders that respond to behavioral therapy generally show the greatest benefit from treatment compared with disorders less likely to respond to behavioral therapy, in part because improvement is easier to measure. In young children with simple phobia, enuresis, and encopresis, noncompliant behaviors respond more effectively to behavioral therapy. *(Ref. 2, pp. 330–331; Ref. 3, pp. 1005–1009)*

10. (c) Parent and child conflicts and relationship problems may be a part of the reason for inpatient care but, by themselves, they are insufficient to meet criteria for hospitalization. The psychiatric disorder should be of sufficient severity to cause significant impairment. Less restrictive treatment settings should have been considered and found inappropriate because of previous failure, lack of motivation, resistance, lack of safety, or unavailability in the patient's region. The most common precipitating factors for inpatient admission are danger to self or danger to others. *(Ref. 2, pp. 340–341; Ref. 3, pp. 1093–1094)*

11. (d) Rapid growth in proprietary psychiatric hospital admissions resulted in closer scrutiny by third-party payers and licensing agencies, and the subsequent reduction of length of hospital stay that was also accompanied by controversy and criticism. All the other reasons listed account for the rapid expansion of for-profit private proprietary psychiatric hospitals since the early 1990s. *(Ref. 3, p. 1093)*

12. (c) An "if...then" approach was also proposed by Jellinek and Herzog. If the last round of diagnostic tests used to rule out medical conditions is negative, then the psychiatric consultation referral should be discussed even if the family is resistant. *(Ref. 3, p. 1401)*

13. (a) Evaluators should obtain information from multiple sources, including other clinicians and care providers. Everyone's information should be taken into consideration during the evaluation. Establishing good rapport and alliance with the patient and caregivers can be helpful. *(Ref. 3, p. 1105)*

14. (d) Partial hospitalization is an ambulatory, multimodal, half-day or full-day (3 to 8 hours per day, 5 days a week) treatment program that is an alternative to inpatient care. Day treatment is the most widely utilized form. *(Ref. 3, pp. 1083–1084)*

15. (e) Acute, immediate, or imminent suicidal ideation, especially when accompanied by specific plans, should be carefully considered in evaluating an appropriate level of care. When there is an active plan for suicide, day treatment usually does not offer sufficient protection. In addition to the goals listed, another goal of day treatment is to support and maintain patients to avoid their long-term hospitalization. *(Ref. 2, pp. 343–344; Ref. 3, p. 1085)*

16. (b) It is important for patients to spend the shortest possible time in treatment, receiving appropriate interventions and reaching maximum benefits. *(Ref. 3, p. 1088)*

17. (d) Younger children show greater benefits than do older ones. Family functioning is a major factor in improvement, and poorer outcomes are associated with patients' disruptive behaviors, patient and family history of mental health treatment, and family separations. *(Ref. 3, pp. 1089–1090)*

18. (a) Group homes are usually smaller than other residential facilities, and, owing to short-term placements and premature termination, often have a short average length of stay. Group homes have fewer staff members per patient and are designed to take less disturbed patients, but more disturbed children are increasingly being placed in them. They are more like a typical living environment than institutional therapeutic settings. *(Ref. 3, p. 1395)*

19. (b) As the responsible physician, a child psychiatrist does not usually take full responsibility for the treatment of the patients in most residential treatment facilities; instead, he or she acts more often as a consultant and a collaborator. *(Ref. 3, pp. 1100–1101)*

20. (c) Protocols for home visitations are not included in the protocols and procedures for psychotropic medication management. *(Ref. 3, pp. 1101–1102)*

15

SPECIAL TOPICS
(CONSULTATION, FORENSICS,
AND PUBLIC HEALTH)

QUESTIONS

Directions: Select the best response for each of the questions 1–29.

1. Which of the following describes the 1979 *Parham* decision regarding the hospitalization of minors?
   a. The adversarial system is the best mechanism for discovering the truth in psychiatric decisions.
   b. Substantive procedural protection should be available to minors.
   c. Parents are presumed to act in their children's best interests and should be free to decide without state interference.
   d. Informed consent is necessary prior to hospitalization.
   e. All children should undergo formal postcommitment review procedures.

2. The result of litigation involving managed care is *best* represented by which of the following statements?
   a. The insurer is liable if, as a result of denial, patient care is compromised.
   b. The utilization review organization is liable if it recommends discharge and patient care is compromised.
   c. The patient is liable for compromised patient care if he or she does not appeal a denial.
   d. The physician is liable for compromised patient care if he or she does not vigorously appeal a denial.
   e. The managed-care organization is ultimately responsible for compromised patient care.

3. The approximate mean prevalence rate of psychiatric disorder among children and adolescents in community populations is:
   a. 5%
   b. 10%
   c. 15%
   d. 30%
   e. 40%

4. Primary prevention refers to which of the following activities?
   a. Rehabilitation
   b. Treatment
   c. Early identification
   d. Early intervention
   e. Onset prevention

5. All of the following statements describe correctly the alternate classification system focusing on intervention *except:*
   a. There are three types of programs: universal, targeted, and clinical.
   b. There are two subtypes in the target program: indicated and selective.
   c. The advantage of the target program is that there is no stigmatization.
   d. The disadvantage of the universal program is that there are no distinctions of high- and low-risk groups.
   e. The advantage of the clinical approach is that it focuses clearly on children with disorders.

6. Public Law 94-142 provides for which of the following?
   a. Mental health care for all children in public schools
   b. An individualized education plan (IEP) for each student
   c. The right of children with a variety of handicaps to an appropriate education
   d. Due process in court hearings involving children
   e. Procedural protection in court commitments

7. In the juvenile justice system, the issue on which the mental health professional's opinion is *most* frequently sought is:
   a. Competency
   b. Insanity
   c. Diminished capacity
   d. Amenability to treatment
   e. Liability

8. The *Tarasoff I* decision refers to:
   a. The duty to hold dangerous patients in the hospital
   b. The duty to ensure patient confidentiality
   c. The duty to hold suicidal patients in the hospital
   d. The duty to obtain informed consent
   e. The duty to warn an endangered third party

9. The *most* frequent reason for malpractice suits being brought against psychiatrists is:
   a. Breach of confidentiality
   b. Improper evaluation for special education
   c. Drug reactions or side effects
   d. Overuse or underuse of psychotropic medications
   e. Failure to report cases of sexual or physical abuse

10. General psychological reactions of children to medical illness and hospitalization include all of the following *except:*
    a. Decreased attachment behavior
    b. Regression
    c. Disturbances in sleep and appetite
    d. Feelings of helplessness
    e. Irritability

11. Identification of pathological or "morbid" grief reactions in parents of children who die of sudden infant death syndrome (SIDS) include all of the following symptoms *except:*
    a. Delayed mourning
    b. Overactivity without a sense of loss

c. Furious hostility

d. Guilty feeling related to perceived negligence

e. Alteration in relationships with friends and family

12. All of the following characteristics are commonly seen in mothers of children diagnosed as having the Munchausen syndrome by proxy *except:*

a. They have had prior extensive exposure to the health-care system.

b. They have difficulty getting along with the hospital staff.

c. They are extremely attentive to the needs of their children.

d. They appear to be comfortable with medical uncertainties.

e. They are always at the hospital when their children are hospitalized.

13. Legal considerations in the psychiatric hospitalization of children and adolescents that are noteworthy, as compared with adult psychiatric hospitalization, include all of the following *except:*

a. Patient age and vulnerability

b. Conflict of a child's rights with those of the parents and society

c. Procedural formality and commitment criteria

d. The nature of the psychiatric disorder

e. The gender of the patient

14. Which of the following is *not* one of the four basic moral principles guiding medical research and health care?

a. Objectivity

b. Autonomy

c. Nonmaleficence

d. Beneficence

e. Justice

15. Basic medical responsibilities to consider with regard to the hospitalization of minors include all of the following *except:*

a. Risks versus benefits

b. Least restrictive alternative

c. Course of treatment

d. Profits for the hospital

e. Adverse effects secondary to being institutionalized

16. Which of the following conditions is *least* likely to have a genetic component?

a. Posttraumatic stress disorder (PTSD)

b. Autism

c. Bipolar disorder

d. Schizophrenia

e. Attention-deficit hyperactivity disorder (ADHD)

17. Which of the following conditions is *least* likely to be affected by biological risk factors compared to the other conditions listed?

a. Early onset schizophrenia

b. Autism

c. Tourette's disorder

d. Obsessive–compulsive disorder (OCD)

e. Adjustment disorder

18. All of the following statements regarding early childhood education accurately represent the current state of our knowledge *except:*

a. Early childhood education does not seem to raise IQ permanently.

b. Sensory learning should precede symbolic learning.

c. Young children learn best through formal instruction.

d. The critical issue in early childcare is not whether the parent is the caregiver, but rather the quality of the childcare.

e. There are pros and cons for universal preschool.

19. The Yale Child Study Center Model for a school mental-health program, developed by James Comer, is *best* described by which of the following statements?

a. It provides for early identification of at-risk children and their involvement in intensive goal-directed interventions.

b. Teachers receive mental health education courses.

c. Seminars in behavior management are provided to school staff members.

d. A systems approach is taken whereby parents are actively involved in school activities.

e. The parents are mostly from middle-class families.

20. The young people seen in juvenile court clinics in recent times appear to be more violent, more disturbed, and less amenable to superficial therapeutic interventions than in the past. Possible reasons for this include all of the following *except:*

a. Decreasing transfer of serious offenders to adult court

b. A clear increase in the incidence of serious juvenile crime

c. Removal of status offenders (children charged with non-criminal misbehavior) from the court's delinquency jurisdiction

d. Provision of due-process protection in juvenile delinquency proceedings

e. Widening of the court's jurisdiction

21. In order to substantiate malpractice, the plaintiff must establish, by a preponderance of the evidence, all of the following elements *except:*

a. The establishment of a physician–patient relationship

b. The physician breaching the duty of care

c. The patient sustaining compensable injury or harm

d. The intention to cause a harm or injury

e. Direct causal relationship

22. All of the following statements regarding legal liability accurately reflect the law *except:*

a. Psychiatrists are legally responsible for the negligent actions of their employees and supervisees.

b. The psychiatrist is expected to carry out his or her fiduciary duty.

c. If a patient offers his or her own mental health as evidence in litigation, the patient waives privilege concerning the specific issue in evidence.

d. As a part of a legal case, a child custody evaluation may be excluded from confidentiality and privilege.

e. A subpoena requires that a psychiatrist testify in court about confidential matters.

23. All of the following must be included in a physician's discussion with a patient (and usually the patient's family when minors are involved) to be considered an informed consent *except:*

a. The nature of the condition requiring intervention

b. Other indications of the proposed treatment

c. The benefits of the treatment and likelihood of success

d. The potential risks and adverse consequence resulting from the treatment

e. The outcome of being or not being treated with the proposed intervention

24. All of the following statements regarding the consent to treatment of children and adolescents represent current legal opinion *except:*

a. Parents who refuse to allow necessary treatments of their children because of their religious convictions are still found liable.

b. In many states, minors themselves can consent to the treatment of certain conditions, such as venereal disease and alcoholism.

c. If a minor can consent to treatment, he or she can also refuse treatment.

d. A parent is not liable for the cost of medical care for a minor unless the parent consented to the treatment.

e. A treating physician should inform the parents of the patient's venereal disease treatment status.

25. Young children, lacking a better explanation for the cause of their illness, may use all of the following explanations *except:*

a. Immanent justice

b. Contagion

c. Misdeeds that led to punishment

d. The interaction of multiple causes

e. Assumption of guilt

26. Reasons why children may fail to report information about illness include all of the following *except:*

a. Grandiosity

b. Egocentrism

c. Magical thinking

d. Shame

e. Fears of retribution

27. All of the following statements regarding the emotional reactions of parents to their premature babies accurately reflect what we know from the current literature *except:*

a. Parents perceive their babies as weaker.

b. Parents interact more with their premature infants.

c. Maternal anxiety level increases after delivery and the baby's coming home.

d. There is a delay in bonding between the baby and mother.

e. Mothers are more likely to overprotect their babies.

28. All of the following are categories of problems faced by the families with children and adolescents who are diagnosed with cancer *except:*

a. Feelings of powerlessness

b. Fixation on family structural hierarchy

c. Changes in family priorities

d. Coping issues

e. Support issues

29. According to Frager and Shapiro (1998), all of the following guidelines are recommended in managing pain in the pediatric population *except:*

a. Pharmacological intervention should be limited.

b. Pain should be considered as an emergency.

c. Different aspects of pain (physiologic, emotional, and social) should be addressed.

d. A physician should be vigilant to pain related to treatment.

e. Pain and treatment effectiveness should be reassessed throughout treatment.

ANSWERS AND EXPLANATIONS

1. **(c)** The *Parham* decision stated that parents are presumed to act in their children's best interests and should be free to decide without state interference, provided there is an independent medical review with the power to deny admission. *(Ref. 1, pp. 911–912; Ref. 3, p. 1285)*

2. **(d)** None of the cases heard have absolved the provider of the responsibility to protest adverse utilization review or insurance denial vigorously when he or she feels patient care may be compromised. Failure to do so has resulted in decisions against the provider. *(Ref. 1, p. 913; Ref. 3, p. 1445; R. D. Geraty, R. L. Hendren, and C. J. Flaa, Ethical perspective on managed care as it relates to child and adolescent psychiatry. JAACAP 31:398–402, 1992)*

3. **(c)** The mean prevalence rate of psychiatric disorder among young people in community samples is 15.8%. *(Ref. 3, p. 1321)*

4. **(e)** Primary prevention programs include interventions designed to reduce the incidence of a particular disorder in a target population. Primary prevention starts before initiation of a disorder, and prevents onset of the disorder. Secondary prevention includes early identification and treatment of a disorder after its onset in order to alter the expression of the pathologic process. Tertiary prevention refers to rehabilitation efforts to minimize the severity of the disorder and promote remission and recovery. *(Ref. 3, p. 1321)*

5. **(c)** An advantage of a universal program is there is no labeling or stigmatization, which is one of the disadvantages of a target program. The advantage of a target program is that it addresses issues early if they are identified accurately. The advantage of a clinical program is that it focuses on children with disorders, but the children have to be referred for services due to lack of an active outreach component. *(Ref. 3, p. 1326)*

6. **(c)** Public Law 94-142 establishes the right of children with various handicaps to an appropriate education and to the "related services" that are needed for the child to benefit from that education. The evaluation involved leads to an IEP for each qualified student. *(Ref. 1, pp. 359, 921; Ref. 3, pp. 582, 1370–1371)*

7. **(d)** In contrast to the adult criminal justice system, instead of being frequently asked for an opinion on issues of competency, insanity, and diminished capacity, the mental professional in the juvenile justice system is frequently asked to address issues related to amenability to treatment. *(Ref. 3, p. 1291)*

8. **(e)** The *Tarasoff I* decision resulted in a ruling that a treating clinician bears a duty to warn threatened persons of foreseeable danger arising from a patient's condition. A subsequent appellate court in *Tarasoff II* modified the duty to that of a duty to protect the foreseeable victim. *(Ref. 1, p. 910; Ref. 3, pp. 1299–1300)*

9. **(c)** While all of the options listed represent potential legal liability, drug reactions or side effects, especially in patients who develop tardive dyskinesia, represent the most frequent cause of malpractice suits against psychiatrists. *(Ref. 3, pp. 1296–1298, 1304)*

10. **(a)** In addition to the other reactions listed, common reactions of children to illness and hospitalization include malaise, pain, increased attachment behavior, regression in bowel and bladder control, feelings of powerlessness, frightening fantasies about illness and procedures, anxiety and mobilization of defenses, and precipitation or aggravation of premorbid psychiatric symptoms. *(Ref. 3, p. 1113)*

11. **(d)** Guilty feelings related to perceived negligence are among a family's normative grief reactions to SIDS. In addition to those listed, other indications of pathologic grief reactions are loss of reality testing and agitated depression. *(Ref. 3, p. 1130)*

12. **(b)** Munchausen syndrome by proxy in children is a disorder wherein a person, usually the mother, fabricates symptoms of illness on behalf of her child. The mother often has previous medical or nursing experience or an extensive history of illness, she is nearly always considered exemplary in all her interactions with hospital staff members, she is always at the hospital, and she appears less worried about her child's illness than is the medical staff. *(Ref. 3, p. 1224)*

13. **(e)** Gender of the patient is usually not a legal consideration in this matter. A child or adolescent may be confined at the request of a parent or guardian in most states. It is often only the admitting physician who stands between the parents' and the child's interests. The commitment of children and adolescents to a psychiatric hospital may represent a conflict of the child's rights to liberty and self-determination with the rights, responsibilities, and duties of the parents and society. The procedural formality and commitment criteria for children are less formal and precise than for adults. Children are more likely to be hospitalized for a "behavioral disorder" than for an acute or severe mental illness, which is not the case with adults. *(Ref. 1, pp. 991–992; Ref. 3, pp. 1285–1288)*

14. **(a)** Objectivity is not one of the four basic moral principles (which include autonomy, nonmaleficence, beneficence, and justice) guiding physicians in their medical research and health care. *(Ref. 3, p. 1442)*

15. **(d)** Issues related to profits for the hospital are not among the basic medical considerations for hospitalizing minors. On the other hand, the physician must consider how hospitalization will affect the child's life over a period of years in terms of disrupted relationships, identity formation, and removal from and return to the home, to name a few. The potential adverse effects secondary to being institutionalized should be considered. Other, less restrictive treatment alternatives must first be considered and deemed inappropriate or unavailable. The course of treatment must be monitored to ensure that the child spends the least amount of time necessary in the hospital. *(Ref. 1, pp. 1066–1067; Ref. 3, pp. 1287–1289)*

16. **(a)** Compared to the other conditions listed, PTSD is least likely to have a genetic component but biological vulnerability to stress is increasingly appreciated as a vulnerability to PTSD. In addition to psychosocial and environmental influences, genetic factors play a significant role in the etiology of a number of mental disorders in children. Some of these disorders, including autism, ADHD, bipolar disorder, and schizophrenia, have very high genetic inheritability. *(Ref. 3, p. 1325)*

17. **(e)** Biological factors may or may not play a role in the etiology of adjustment disorder. However, biological factors certainly play significant roles in early onset schizophrenia, pervasive developmental disorder (PDD), autism, Tourette's disorder, social phobia, and OCD. *(Ref. 3, p. 1325)*

18. **(c)** Infants and young children are eager to learn from their own explorations, needing to acquire the basics of the world before they can learn the symbolic world through formal instruction. There is no evidence that early childhood education permanently raises a child's IQ. When a child is cared for by an experienced, warm adult (with one adult caring for not more than three infants), and the environment is a safe, pleasant, and interesting one, there is no evidence of lasting untoward effects of day care as compared with home/maternal care. There is a need for universal preschool in the United States, although there are challenges regarding how to set up a quality, affordable, and accessible preschool education program. *(Ref. 3, pp. 1249–1251)*

19. **(d)** The Yale Model applies a systems approach to school problems and focuses on improving the school's social environment by (1) encouraging parent participation through a parent program in support of school activities, (2) integrating the arts and athletic programs into the school's activities, and (3) establishing a multidisciplinary mental health team to provide consultation on the management of student behavior problems. These activities are coordinated by a representative governing body composed of administrators, teachers, support staff, and parents. Parents and students in this study are from poor families in the inner city of New Haven, Connecticut. *(Ref. 3, pp. 1256–1258)*

20. **(e)** Since the 1960s, the procedural protection for juveniles was mandated, and the court's jurisdiction was narrowed. Due-process restrictions on the transfer of serious offenders to adult courts have led to an increase in the number of violent youth being seen in juvenile court. Status offenders (children charged with noncriminal misbehavior) are no longer permitted to be confined in juvenile correctional facilities, in essence removing them from the court's jurisdiction. While this has removed some youth from the juvenile courts, it has left more disturbed young people there. *(Ref. 3, pp. 1290–1291)*

21. **(d)** The term malpractice refers to *unintentional* wrongful behavior by a professional practitioner in the course of professional duty that results in a harm or an injury to a patient or client, which is secondary to a failure to exercise a reasonable degree of prudence, diligence, knowledge, or skill. Four "Ds," including duty, dereliction, damage, and direct, are commonly used to describe the essential elements for the plaintiff to establish a malpractice case. *(Ref. 1, p. 912; Ref. 3, p. 1293)*

22. **(e)** A subpoena requires only that the clinician appear in court and does not compel the clinician to testify about confidential matters. A supervisor is legally liable for the actions of his or her supervisees or employees. Fiduciary duty refers to the physician's duty to act in the patient's best interests. In psychiatry, breaches of fiduciary trust include improper sexual contact, invasion of privacy, outrageous manipulation of the patient's emotions, and the use of patients for financial gain. There are some exceptions of privilege and confidentiality. *(Ref. 3, pp. 1293–1294)*

23. **(b)** It is not necessary to discuss other indications of the proposed intervention. Most case decisions indicate that the physician should discuss all the other matters listed with the patient (and possibly the family, depending on the state and on the age of the minor), and also the available alternatives (including their risks and consequences) to the proposed treatment. *(Ref. 3, p. 1297)*

24. **(e)** Most states do not allow physicians to reveal youths' status of venereal disease treatment to their parents. The age at which most states allow a minor to consent to a treatment is 16, although in some states it is 14 years of age. The mature minor rule refers to the principle that if a minor understands the nature of a proposed treatment and its risks, and if the treatment does not involve serious risks, the young person can give valid consent. *(Ref. 3, pp. 1305–1306)*

25. **(d)** It is not until children are about 12 or 13 years old that they begin to appreciate that illness involves multiple causes that are the result of the host and the environment. Younger children are likely to resort to explanations of illness that attribute it to immanent justice or the belief that natural justice can emanate from inanimate objects, where misdeeds will be punished, leading to guilt and shame. Preoperational children usually overextend the concept of contagion to include non-contagious illness. *(Ref. 3, pp. 1120–1121)*

26. **(a)** Grandiosity is not one of the common reasons why children fail to report their symptoms. Egocentrism and magical thinking are common in young children. They assume that if they do not wish to be ill, then they will not be ill, or that vocalizing symptoms will make their fears reality. Children who use immanent-justice explanations for illness may not vocalize their symptoms because of shame and the fear of retribution. *(Ref. 3, p. 1121)*

27. **(b)** Parents of premature infants interact far less with their "sick" infants than do parents of well babies. Parents of premature babies tend to experience anxiety, overprotect their children, and experience delayed bonding and attachment. *(Ref. 3, pp. 1124–1125)*

28. **(b)** Changing of family dynamics (not fixation on family hierarchy) is one of the eight categories of problems faced by parents with youth suffering from cancer. In addition to the others listed, being governed by the illness, dealing with the reactions of others, and quality of life are problems parents face under these circumstances. *(Ref. 3, p. 1139)*

29. **(a)** Both nonpharmacological and pharmacological interventions should be used. In addition to the other guidelines listed, involvement of the parents and entire family is recommended. *(Ref. 3, p. 1140)*

16

RESEARCH DESIGN, STATISTICS, AND TECHNOLOGIES

QUESTIONS

Directions: Select the best response for each of the questions 1–23.

1. All of the following statements regarding reliability and validity are accurate *except:*

   a. The validity of an instrument refers to the extent to which it measures what it was intended to measure.
   b. Reliability refers to the extent to which results obtained with an instrument can be reproduced.
   c. Validity ensures reliability.
   d. Test–retest reliability is a strenuous test of interrater reliability.
   e. Validity includes predictive validity, face validity, and construct validity.

2. Randomized experimental research designs are usually preferred over quasi-experimental designs because they:

   a. Are easier to execute
   b. Eliminate bias
   c. Are less expensive to carry out
   d. Have one active independent variable
   e. Require little training to perform

3. All of the following statements regarding the Diagnostic Interview Schedule for Children (DISC) are accurate *except:*

   a. It is a semistructured interview.
   b. It is designed to provide a DSM-IV diagnosis.
   c. It can be administered by lay interviewers with training.
   d. It is very sensitive, but has lower specificity.
   e. It has high test–retest reliability in diagnosing simple phobia.

4. Which of the following statements regarding associational research designs and data analysis is *incorrect?*

   a. They are designed to examine the relationship between two continuous variables.
   b. Variables can be both independent and dependent.
   c. Coefficient *r* expresses the Pearson product moment correlation.
   d. A strong positive relationship is found if $r > 0.5$.
   e. The *r* can be expressed with degrees of freedom and significance level.

5. Which of the following represents statistical significance?

   a. The *p* value
   b. The *r* value
   c. The *K* value
   d. The *d* score
   e. The X^2 value

6. All of the following statements regarding logistic regression analysis and discriminant analysis are correct *except:*

   a. Logistic regression requires fewer assumptions than discriminant analysis, and performs better.
   b. Logistic regression estimates the probability an event will occur.
   c. The coefficient is expressed as an odds score in logistic regression.
   d. An odds ratio (the ratio of two odds, OR) is essential to logistic regression.
   e. OR = 0 means random association.

7. Which of the following neuroimaging techniques is *best* suited to studying developmental brain abnormalities in children?

   a. Computed tomography (CT)
   b. Magnetic resonance imaging (MRI)
   c. Positron-emission tomography (PET)
   d. Magnetoencephalography (MEG)
   e. Single-photon emission computed tomography (SPECT)

8. Magnetic resonance spectroscopy (MRS) can be used to measure all of the following *except:*

   a. Energy metabolism
   b. Amino acids
   c. Cell membrane stability
   d. Cerebral blood flow
   e. Neurotransmitters

9. All of the following statements regarding SPECT are accurate *except:*

   a. It is capable of monitoring brain activity.
   b. It provides clear spatial resolution of white matter changes.
   c. It is capable of measuring neurotransmitter activity.
   d. It is relatively inexpensive compared to PET.
   e. Radiation exposure is a potential limitation.

10. All of the following are the advantages of interviewer-based interviews compared to respondent-based interviews *except:*

    a. Being conducted and coded properly
    b. Cross-checking discrepancies
    c. Using open-ended questions
    d. Less prone to overdiagnosing
    e. Less intensive training required

11. In recent years, newer neuroimaging technologies have been applied to the research of pediatric brain development. All of the following statements regarding the differences in neurological development in children born prematurely compared to those born full-term are correct *except:*

a. If there is not a complicated neonatal course, children born prematurely have a similar IQ compared to children born at term.

b. More than half of children born prematurely require special assistance in school.

c. MRI shows reduction of cortical gray matter and white matter in children born prematurely.

d. MRI shows increased CSF volume in children born prematurely.

e. MRI shows reduced volumes in sensorimotor, parieto-occipital, subgenual cortices, basal ganglia, amygdala, hippocampus, and corpus callosum.

12. Which of the following statements regarding the type II error is correct?

a. Null hypothesis is not rejected when it is true.

b. Null hypothesis is rejected when it is false.

c. Null hypothesis is not rejected when it is false.

d. Null hypothesis is rejected when it is true.

e. The alternative hypothesis is rejected when it is false.

13. Which of the following statements regarding sensitivity and specificity is *incorrect*?

a. Sensitivity is the percentage of negative results among individuals who do not have the disease for which they are being tested.

b. Sensitivity is important when trying to identify as many cases as possible.

c. Sensitivity is the percentage of positive results among individuals who have the disease for which they are being tested.

d. Specificity is the percentage of negative test results in patients who actually do not have the disease.

e. Specificity is important in trying to include only true cases.

14. Changing the threshold that separates children into "disordered" and "not disordered" can have a noticeable effect on the prevalence and comorbidity of the disorder. All of the following affect thresholds *except:*

a. Altering the pool of symptoms used to measure the disorder

b. Gender of the patients

c. Changing the number or severity of symptoms required

d. Modifying the criteria needed for associated impairments

e. Showing the independent evidence of impairment for children above the threshold

15. All of the following statements regarding the Schedule for Affective Disorders and Schizophrenia for School-Age Children (K-SADS) are accurate *except:*

a. It is a semistructured interview.

b. It gives a DSM-IV diagnosis.

c. It requires little training to administer.

d. It is highly specific, but may have low sensitivity.

e. It is a downward extension of adult SADS.

16. All of the following statements regarding functional magnetic resonance imaging (fMRI) are accurate *except:*

a. It identifies brain activity while the subject performs a cognitive task.

b. The image intensity changes result from the variable oxygenation levels in the regions of interest.

c. Its spatial and temporal resolutions are superior to those of conventional PET and SPECT.

d. Its temporal resolution is superior to that of the electroencephalograph (EEG).

e. It is relatively safe in children.

17. All of the following statements regarding diffusion tensor imaging (DTI) are correct *except:*

a. It is an application of MRI technology.

b. It has a unique strength in providing information about the orientation and integrity of gray matter tracts.

c. It is based on T1 and T2 relaxation times to produce the images.

d. Initially it was used to diagnose stroke.

e. There are potential uses for studying brain connectivity.

18. All of the following are essential elements of information that should be transmitted to research subjects during the informed consent process *except:*

a. Purpose and duration of the research

b. Foreseeable risks and benefits

c. Confidentiality of records

d. Contact information in case of questions

e. Specifying loss of benefits due to refusal to participate

19. Which of the following is *most* essential to be obtained from child subjects before they participate in clinical research?

a. Assent

b. Permission

c. Consent

d. Authorization

e. Acceptance

20. All of the following statements regarding the developmental changes in the EEG are accurate *except:*

a. There are both qualitative and quantitative maturational and developmental changes in the EEG.

b. Between the ages of about 5 and 11 years, EEG changes have been characterized by an increase in slower frequencies, and a decrease in higher frequencies.

c. At the age of 4 years, there is a developmental peak of theta activity.

d. Occipital alpha rhythm increases progressively from infancy to adulthood.

e. Increased complexity of EEG with age correlates with the increased complexity of brain activity with maturation.

21. Which of the following statements regarding MEG is *most* accurate?

a. It detects signals representing a direct index of neuronal activity.

b. It is relatively simple and inexpensive.

c. The clinical yield in child psychiatry has been impressive.

d. It has been widely utilized in studying adults.

e. It measures not only cerebral blood flow but also blood oxygenation.

22. Data from all of the following studies can be used to support a genetic component in the development of attention-deficit hyperactivity disorder (ADHD) *except:*

a. Twin studies

b. Sibling and half-sibling studies

c. Environmental toxicological studies

d. Adoption studies

e. Family studies

23. A region was identified as a dyslexia susceptibility region through a genome-wide linkage study in a large extended Norwegian family on which of the following chromosomes?

a. Chromosome 1

b. Chromosome 2

c. Chromosome 5

d. Chromosome 11

e. Chromosome 18

ANSWERS AND EXPLANATIONS

1. **(c)** Validity does not guarantee reliability, just as reliability cannot ensure validity. Validity may include predictive validity, face validity, and construct validity, whereas reliability may include test–retest reliability and interrater reliability. Interitem consistency is also used to estimate reliability. *(Ref. 1, pp. 139–140; Ref. 3, pp. 501, 557–558)*

2. **(b)** In contrast to the quasi-experimental studies, subjects in randomized studies are assigned randomly to groups (experimental or control), with an advantage of eliminating bias. Single and double blinding further reduces the possibility of bias. This leads to providing more convincing evidence that the independent variable rather than the dependent or control variable caused the difference. Both and experimental designs require an active variable. *(G. A. Morgan, J. A. Gliner, and R. J. Harmon: Randomized experimental designs. JAACAP, 39:1062–1063, 2000)*

3. **(a)** The DISC is a highly structured instrument where the wording of the questions must be followed closely. Because of this, trained laypersons can administer the interview and few cases are missed (highly sensitive), but some diagnoses that are made are false positives (low specificity). The kappa value is 0.86 in diagnosing simple phobia—a high level of reliability, when combining both parent and child interviews. *(Ref. 1, pp. 104, 142–143; Ref. 3, pp. 547–549)*

4. **(b)** In associational research designs, the two variables are either independent or dependent. The Pearson product moment correlation is used to estimate the strength of association between the two variables, and expresses as coefficient r, ranging from -1 to $+1$, with value > 0.5, indicating a strong positive association. *(J. A. Gliner, G.A. Morgan, and R. J. Harmon: Basic associational designs: analysis and interpretation, JAACAP, 41:1256–1258, 2002)*

5. **(a)** The p value represents the strength of correlation between two variables, indicating the probability an outcome could occur if the null hypothesis were true. Statistical significance should not be interpreted as clinical significance or approval of the null hypothesis. The K value represents the correlation coefficient of reliability. The X^2 represents the chi-square value. The r family, d family, and the measures of risk potency are proposed measures of sample size. *(H. C. Kraemer et al.: Measures of clinical significance, JAACAP, 42:1524–1529, 2003)*

6. **(e)** An OR = 1 (not = 0) or odds = 0 indicates a random association. Discriminant analysis requires more assumptions than logistic regression analysis does to make an optimal prediction. The odds are used to express the probability an event will occur in logistic regression, and the odds ratio increases with an increase of a positive association, and decreases with a negative association. *(G. A. Morgan, J. J. Vaske, J. A. Gliner, and R. J. Harmon: Logistic regression and discriminant analysis: Use and interpretation, JAACAP, 42:994–997, 2003)*

7. **(b)** Both MRI and MEG are ideally suited to study structural, physiologic, and developmental brain abnormalities in children and to perform repeated measures, since they involve no ionizing radiation or radioactive isotopes and have been shown to have an absence of biologic hazards at currently used field strengths. However, MRI is more extensively developed and studied than is MEG. The use of CT exposes the child to x-rays, and PET exposes the child to radiation. Although SPECT provides for functional neuroimaging, it involves small amounts of radioisotopes. *(Ref. 1, p. 187; Ref. 3, pp. 132–135)*

8. **(d)** The MRS technique has been used to measure amino acids, neurotransmitters, metabolites related to energy production, and metabolism of lipids and carbohydrates. It has not been used to measure cerebral blood flow that can be measured by fMRI. *(Ref. 1, p. 187; Ref. 3, pp. 134–135)*

9. **(b)** The SPECT technique provides a three-dimensional image of brain function. It measures cerebral blood flow and metabolic activity with minimal radiation exposure. Using long-lived isotopes, SPECT is cheaper than PET. The major disadvantages are the limited clinical experience with it and its inferior spatial resolution compared to that of PET. *(Ref. 1, p. 187; Ref. 3, p. 134)*

10. **(e)** Respondent-based interviews require less intensive training with more readiness of designing and using computer-assisted and computer-administered interviews. However, neither of these two types of interviews is an ideal tool for every situation, so their advantages and disadvantages must be considered for each research design. *(Ref. 3, pp. 550–551)*

11. **(a)** Premature infants weigh less than 1500 g, make up about 12 to 32% of neurodevelopmental disturbances, and account for 1.5% of all live new births in the United States. Even without complications during neonatal periods, children born prematurely have an IQ one standard deviation below the norm. MRI techniques facilitate neurodevelopmental research by identifying brain anatomical changes in children born prematurely, some of which correlates with low IQs in this population. *(Ref. 3, pp. 136–137)*

12. **(c)** A type II error refers to incorrectly deciding no difference exists when there really is a difference (the null hypothesis is not rejected when it is false). A type I error refers to deciding a difference exists when there is really no difference (null hypothesis is rejected when it is true). *(J. A. Gliner, G. A. Morgan, and R. J. Harmon: Instruction to inferential statistics and hypothesis testing, JAACAP, 39:1568–1570, 2000)*

13. **(a)** Sensitivity is the proportion of true cases that the test selects. Specificity is the proportion of subjects who do not have the disease in the group that the test identifies as negative. *(Ref. 1, p. 140)*

14. (b) Gender does not seem to affect the threshold. The meaningfulness of a threshold is enhanced if associated data show a discontinuity at the point of the threshold. *(Ref. 3, p. 1322)*

15. (c) The K-SADS is a semistructured interview, meaning that the interviewer is encouraged to follow a certain format, but can modify questions. Because of the semistructured nature of the test, it should be given by a person after training and reliability determination. It does yield a DSM-IV diagnosis. For different testing purposes, several new versions of K-SADS are available, including K-SADS-P, K-SADS-E, K-SADS-PL, WASH-U-K-SADS, and COLUMBIA K-SADS. *(Ref. 1, pp. 142–143, 413; Ref. 3, p. 546)*

16. (d) Compared to fMRI, EEG has a much better temporal resolution than fMRI. However, fMRI has better resolution than PET and SPECT. fMRI can test subjects undertaking cognitive tasks by identifying changes in oxygenation levels of identified regions of interest. *(Ref. 3, p. 134)*

17. (b) DTI specifically focuses on the white matter and evaluates the orientation and integrity of the white matter tracts. DTI images are based on T1 and T2 relaxation times, providing information regarding neuronal connectivity. Clinically, it was first used to diagnose stroke, and then to show the white matter loss in multiple sclerosis, schizophrenia, dyslexia, and preterm birth. *(Ref. 3, pp. 134–135)*

18. (e) According to federal regulations, certain key elements of information must be transmitted to the research subjects during the informed consent process. Participation is on a voluntary basis, and no loss of benefits should result from refusal to participate in research. *(Ref. 3, pp. 1433–1436)*

19. (a) Assent is the term that describes children's agreement to participate in a research project. Informed consent is usually given by parents or legal guardians who have ultimate rights to authorize or refuse participation. Permission refers to the collective decision and judgment of the family in deciding to allow the child to participate. *(Ref. 3, pp. 1436–1437)*

20. (b) Between the ages of about 5 and 11 years, EEG changes have been characterized by a *decrease* in slower frequencies, and an *increase* in higher frequencies. In addition to the other changes in EEG listed, many studies also show that change patterns of alpha activity throughout child and adolescent development coincide with brain development in youth measured by other means, such as brain weight, head circumference, cortical thickness, neuronal density, and pyramidal cell dimensions. *(Ref. 3, pp. 61–62)*

21. (a) Magnetoencephalography is a technique combining both magnetic field and EEG techniques, detecting signals that represent a direct index of neuronal activities. In contrast, most other neuroimaging methods (for example, fMRI) detect indirect indices of neuronal activities by measuring cerebral blood flow and oxygenation. *(Ref. 3, p. 123)*

22. (c) Data from twin, sibling and half-sibling, adoption, and family studies suggest genetic factors that play a role in the development of ADHD. Toxicological studies support environmental influence on the development of ADHD. *(Ref. 3, pp. 370–371)*

23. (b) A genome-wide linkage study was done in a large extended Norwegian family, and a dyslexia susceptibility region was identified on the short arm of chromosome 2. Linkage studies have been performed on children with several psychiatric disorders with mixed and, frequently, difficult to replicate results (even in those with very high inheritability, such as autism and ADHD), indicating an unlikely single gene involvement in any of the common psychiatric disorders. *(Ref. 3, pp. 418–423)*

PART II
MOCK EXAMINATION

The oral portion of the Child and Adolescent Board Examination consists of three written and/or videotaped vignettes (preschool-age child, school-age child, and a consultation) and one live adolescent patient who is interviewed by the candidate. Each segment is followed by a 30-minute discussion by the candidate with the examiners. The format requires that the candidate gather, process, and organize information quickly and efficiently, and articulate a coherent presentation under pressure. The candidate must identify the important clinical information given and that which is still needed, and put together a formulation, differential diagnosis, treatment plan, and prognosis. In doing this, the candidate should demonstrate competence in biologic, developmental, psychological, and social realms.

It is often helpful for the candidate to arrange for a practice or mock oral examination prior to the actual examination. The questions in this section cover the essential elements of the oral examination, and offer examples of types of questions that the examiners might expect to have answered.

17

CLINICAL ASSESSMENT, DIFFERENTIAL DIAGNOSIS, FORMULATION, AND TREATMENT PLANNING

QUESTIONS

Directions: Select the best response for each of the questions 1–35.

1. All of the following are examples of the clinical process of the interview, as opposed to the clinical content of the interview, *except:*

   a. It elucidates the child's emotional reactions to the subjects being discussed.
   b. It refers to the actual verbal exchange.
   c. It may be evidenced by play interruptions.
   d. It may be evidenced through body language.
   e. It includes the interviewer's own emotional reactions.

2. Certain techniques of gathering information from and communicating with patients are frequently used, while others are best used infrequently. Of the following techniques, which one should be used *cautiously* with children and their families?

   a. Open-ended questions
   b. Summation
   c. Reflection
   d. Clarification
   e. Interpretation

3. Which of the following techniques of communications is likely to be the *most* effective when gathering a thorough history from an adolescent patient?

   a. Exclusive use of open-ended questions
   b. Explicit approaches and direct questions about the adolescent's life
   c. Silence until the adolescent feels like talking
   d. Confrontation of inconsistencies and contradictions in the history as they appear
   e. Trying hard to be cool

4. All of the following represent negative effects on the goodness of fit between the primary caregiver and his or her child *except:*

   a. Similar parent and infant temperaments
   b. Poor parenting skills
   c. Low threshold of responsiveness in the child
   d. Environmental stress
   e. A lack of environmental support

5. All of the following are considered neurologic soft signs *except:*

   a. Dysdiadochokinesis
   b. Coordination defects
   c. Dysgraphesthesia
   d. Electroencephalogram (EEG) epileptiform discharges
   e. Motor slowness/inaccuracy

6. All of the following signs and symptoms are usually associated with formal thought disorder in children *except:*

   a. An imaginary companion
   b. Bizarre hallucinations
   c. Illogical thought processes
   d. Significant loosening of association
   e. Delusions of reference

7. Hallucinations that are associated with major depressive disorder in children and adolescents may be distinguished from those associated with schizophrenia by which of the following?

   a. Fragmented and incoherent in nature
   b. Bizarre content
   c. Paranoid quality
   d. Inability to control
   e. Depressive nature

8. A child should be able to draw a symbolic representation of a person consisting of circles and lines by which of the following ages?

   a. 2 to 3 Years
   b. 3 to 4 Years
   c. 5 to 6 Years
   d. 7 to 8 Years
   e. 8 to 10 Years

9. Psychological testing alone is able to do all of the following *except:*

   a. Provide a measure of intelligence
   b. Clarify the nature of the learning disability
   c. Confirm the presence of a thought disorder
   d. Establish a diagnosis
   e. Elucidate depressive symptomatology

10. Conditions known to produce a false positive dexamethasone suppression test (DST) as a measure of depression in children and adolescents include all of the following *except:*

    a. Hypopituitarism
    b. Anorexia nervosa
    c. Barbiturates
    d. Acute alcohol withdrawal
    e. Suicidal ideation

11. Serum amylase determination is used to monitor which of the following conditions seen in children and adolescents?

    a. Wilson's disease
    b. Binging and purging behavior
    c. Acute intermittent porphyria
    d. Alcoholism
    e. Emaciated anorexia nervosa

12. Obtaining an EEG is useful in the evaluation of psychiatric disorders in children and adolescents in all of the following cases *except:*

    a. To help rule out a psychosis
    b. To evaluate "absence" episodes
    c. To evaluate temporal lobe seizures
    d. To evaluate and rule out pseudoseizure
    e. To evaluate complex partial seizures

13. Magnetic resonance imaging (MRI) is preferred to computed tomography (CT) in all of the following conditions *except:*

    a. Demyelinating disorders
    b. Visualization of the temporal lobes
    c. Visualization of midline structures
    d. Visualization of cortical contusion
    e. Location of an aneurysm clip

14. All of the following describe the clinical formulation *except:*

    a. A multidimensional picture of the child or adolescent
    b. A biopsychosocial integration of findings
    c. An integrated summary of interaction of organic and environmental factors and inner conflicts
    d. A full description of the clinical findings
    e. A description of the interaction of all of the important variables leading to the psychiatric disorder and helping to develop a comprehensive treatment plan

15. Which of the following lithium serum levels is the lowest where signs of lithium toxicity typically occur?

    a. 0.2 mEq/L
    b. 0.4 mEq/L
    c. 1.4 mEq/L
    d. 1.6 mEq/L
    e. 2.0 mEq/L

16. Which of the following divalproex (Depakote) levels should be the target serum level in treating juvenile bipolar disorder?

    a. 20 to 60 μg/L
    b. 40 to 80 μg/L
    c. 60 to 100 μg/L
    d. 85 to 110 μg/L
    e. 120 to 150 μg/L

17. In the psychiatric assessment of children and adolescents, parents are often interviewed first or in the presence of the young person. However, the young person can be interviewed first. All of the following are considered appropriate situations for interviewing the young person first *except:*

    a. Unavailability of parents
    b. Confidentiality issues
    c. Adolescent self-referral
    d. Adolescent-patient preference
    e. Very young children

18. In therapy with adolescents, therapist–patient interactions are confidential. In general, the therapist should not disclose specific information to the patient's parents or others without his or her permission. Which of the following is *not* one of the exceptions to this confidentiality rule?

    a. Risk of suicide
    b. Adolescent's preference to let the clinician be a "spokesperson"
    c. All cases of substance use
    d. Risk of homicide
    e. Suspicion of physical or sexual abuse

19. Which of the following statements regarding neurologic soft signs is *inaccurate?*

    a. They often reflect nonspecific neurodevelopmental findings.
    b. They do not reflect a specific neurologic lesion.
    c. They are influenced by heredity.
    d. They predict the diagnosis of attention-deficit hyperactivity disorder (ADHD).
    e. They are likely to be associated with premotor frontal lobe underdevelopment.

20. Which of the following is the *least* likely potential cause of thought disorder in children and adolescents?

    a. Hartnup's disease
    b. Iron deficiency
    c. Metabolic disorders
    d. Drug intoxication
    e. Thyrotoxicosis

21. Infectious illnesses that may give rise to hallucinations include all of the following *except:*

    a. Encephalitis
    b. Acute febrile illnesses
    c. Meningitis
    d. Mononucleosis
    e. Brain abscess

22. Which of the following defense mechanisms is *least* likely to be used by a young child?

    a. Altruism
    b. Externalization
    c. Denial
    d. Regression
    e. Displacement

23. During a psychiatric examination of youth, all of the following are common positive attributes of young people that the clinician should make note of *except:*

    a. Physical attractiveness
    b. Affective lability
    c. Good coping skills
    d. Supportive and stable relationships with others
    e. Realistic self-esteem

24. All of the following steps should be part of the conclusion of the evaluation of a child or adolescent *except:*

a. Informing the patient and the family of what comes next
b. Discussing the recommendations with the child and the family
c. Providing an accounting of the child's and the family's strengths and areas of difficulty
d. Sending a report to the youth's school teacher
e. Enlisting the support of the family for the treatment plan

25. Laboratory tests of thyroid function are *least* useful in the evaluation of which of the following psychiatric symptoms?

    a. Anxiety
    b. Mania
    c. Mental retardation
    d. Psychosis
    e. Panic attacks

26. All of the following statements regarding use of the dexamethasone suppression test (DST) with children and adolescents are accurate *except:*

    a. It has no significant value in screening for depression.
    b. It has a higher sensitivity in inpatients than in outpatients.
    c. Its sensitivity is higher in depressed adolescents than in depressed children.
    d. Its specificity is higher in inpatients than in outpatients.
    e. It may be useful in monitoring response of depression treatment.

27. Genetic karyotyping to determine the chromosome number and morphology is useful in the evaluation of all of the following conditions *except:*

    a. Fragile X syndrome
    b. Turner's syndrome
    c. Klinefelter's syndrome
    d. Wilson's disease
    e. Prader–Willi syndrome

28. Brain imaging such as CT or MRI should be seriously considered to assist diagnosis under all of the following conditions *except:*

    a. ADHD
    b. Abnormal EEG with seizure
    c. Rapid onset of severe psychiatric symptoms
    d. Focal neurologic finding
    e. Certain genetic syndromes

29. All of the following statements regarding the classification system used in the DSM-IV are accurate *except:*

    a. It is a categorical approach.
    b. It is a dimensional approach.
    c. Dimensional classification has more satisfactory reliability.
    d. Categorical classification has been used in all systems of medical diagnosis.

e. DSM-IV should not be used mechanically.

30. Some changes have been made for the following disorders from the DSM-IV to the DSM-IV-TR with the *exception* of:

    a. ADHD
    b. Mental retardation
    c. Rett's disorder
    d. Autistic disorder
    e. Selective mutism

31. The biases that can potentially influence clinical diagnosis include all of the following *except:*

    a. Gathering data selectively
    b. Being systematic in organizing available information
    c. Prematurely making a diagnosis
    d. Assumption of a nonexisting correlation between symptoms and illness
    e. Overinfluence by the expertise of others seeing the child

32. The dynamic portion of the formulation is based on all of the following *except:*

    a. Ego psychological factors
    b. Separation–individuation
    c. Developmental lines
    d. Coherent schemes related to meaning of behavior
    e. Operant conditioning

33. An electrocardiogram (ECG) may be indicated in children and adolescents under all of the following conditions *except:*

    a. Taking tricyclic antidepressants
    b. Taking certain neuroleptics
    c. Taking selective serotonin reuptake inhibitors (SSRIs)
    d. Before initiation of psychotropic medicines with a known cardiac disease history
    e. High cardiac risk before starting psychotropic medicines

34. The medical workup and monitoring for neuroleptic malignant syndrome should include all of the following *except:*

    a. Complete blood count (CBC)
    b. Urine myoglobulin
    c. Creatinine phosphokinase (CPK)
    d. Serum thyroxine (T_4)
    e. Vital signs and mental status

35. The medical workup for anorexia nervosa should include all of the following *except:*

    a. Blood chemistry profile
    b. EEG
    c. CBC
    d. Bone x-rays
    e. EKG

ANSWERS AND EXPLANATIONS

1. **(b)** The content of the clinical interview refers to the actual verbal exchange. The process of the interview is particularly evidenced by the sensitivity and sensibility that evolve "beneath the surface" and "between the lines" of the actual verbal exchange. Process communications are often revealed through play interruption, body language, symbolic reference to past events, avoidance of certain topics, and the interviewer's own emotional reaction. *(R. L. Hendren, Assessment and interviewing strategies for suicidal patients over the life cycle. In S. J. Blumenthal and D. J. Kupfer (Eds.). [1990] Suicide Over the Life Cycle. APA Press, Washington, DC; Ref. 1, pp. 103–105, 113–115; Ref. 3, pp. 525–531)*

2. **(e)** Open-ended questions, summation, reflection, and clarification are all nonintrusive ways of gathering information from the patient; they do not imply undue familiarity and are not likely to result in a defensive or guarded response. Interpretations, on the other hand, can imply what the patient should feel or do, and they suggest value judgments. They should be used cautiously, especially until good rapport has been established. *(R. L. Hendren, Assessment and interviewing strategies for suicidal patients over the life cycle. In S. J. Blumenthal and D. J. Kupfer (Eds.). [1990] Suicide Over the Life Cycle. APA Press, Washington, DC.; Ref. 1, pp. 103–105, 113–115; Ref. 3, pp. 525–531)*

3. **(b)** Adolescents usually respond best to clearly stated questions that are asked directly and explicitly. The exclusive use of indirect and open-ended questions often fails to engage an adolescent, as does silence. Early expressions of sympathy or assumed empathy can appear insincere and condescending, and confrontation often leads to a power struggle. Clinicians should not be phony, deceptive, or overly ingratiating, or try hard to be cool. *(Ref. 1, pp. 113–115; Ref. 3, p. 530)*

4. **(a)** Goodness of fit involves the relationship between the child and the primary caregiver's temperament, the caregiver's parenting skills, and environmental stress and support. A low threshold of responsiveness is associated with the "difficult" temperament cluster. The goodness of fit will depend on the match between the caregiver's temperamental qualities and the infant's temperamental qualities. *(Ref. 1, p. 35; Ref. 2, pp. 10–11; Ref. 3, pp. 221–223)*

5. **(d)** Neurologic soft signs are nonspecific neurologic abnormalities, as opposed to hard neurologic signs, which represent specific neurologic damage, such as EEG epileptiform discharges that indicate seizure. *(Ref. 1, p. 492; Ref. 3, pp. 573–574)*

6. **(a)** The presence of an imaginary companion can be a normal phenomenon in children and is distinguished from a hallucination by its volitional appearance and friendly nature. At times, imaginary companions are present in children with schizotypal disorder. *(Ref. 3, pp. 359–363, 536–537)*

7. **(e)** Hallucinations can be associated with schizophrenia or major depression, and it is often difficult to distinguish between the two in children and adolescents. This accounts in part for the overdiagnosis of schizophrenia and underdiagnosis of bipolar disorder in children and adolescents. Generally, the hallucinations associated with major depressive disorder are nonbizarre, and mood congruent with a depressive content and theme, at times with delusions of guilt and nihilism. *(Ref. 3, pp. 362–364, 536)*

8. **(c)** By 2 to 3 years of age, a child can scribble in a circular motion; by 4 years of age, a child can draw lines; by 5 to 6 years of age, a child can draw a person consisting of circles, ellipses, and lines; and by 7 to 10 years of age, a child can draw a figure with some amount of detail. *(Ref. 3, p. 537)*

9. **(d)** Psychological testing can be helpful in providing a global measure of intelligence and specific learning disabilities, especially when combined with other measures of adaptive functioning. It can also be useful in confirming the presence or absence of a formal thought disorder. Such tests may provide additional information to help establish a diagnosis or treatment plan, but must be combined with other sources of information. *(Ref. 1, pp. 165–168; Ref. 2, pp. 15–19; Ref. 3, pp. 555–556)*

10. **(a)** Conditions that affect the neuroendocrine system can invalidate the DST and should be ruled out before the test is interpreted. Hypopituitarism gives a false negative response to the DST as a measure of depression. The DST does not make a diagnosis; it provides little help with choice of treatment and it does not predict prognosis. Therefore, it is seldom used. *(Ref. 1, p. 450; Ref. 3, pp. 773–774)*

11. **(b)** Baseline serum amylase levels are increased in patients who binge–purge as compared with restricting anorexia nervosa patients. They also increase after binge–purge activity and decrease when binging–purging is discontinued. Serum ceruloplasmin is used to evaluate Wilson's disease; porphobilinogen and aminolevulinic acid are used to evaluate acute intermittent porphyria. Serum amylase is also used in the evaluation of pancreatic disorders that may be associated with alcoholism, but this is not seen in children or adolescents. *(Ref. 1, p. 698; Ref. 3, pp. 694–695)*

12. **(a)** Because of the high prevalence of abnormal EEG findings in the general population and the lack of association of specific findings with specific psychiatric disorders, routine EEGs are not indicated in the workup of psychiatric disorders in children and adolescents, except when there is evidence of seizure disorders. Electroencephalogram under video monitoring is used to differentiate epilepsy seizure from pseudoseizure. *(Ref. 1, p. 187; Ref. 3, pp. 755–758)*

13. **(e)** In general, MRI is preferable to CT, except when looking for calcified tissue and when there are contraindications to the magnetic field, such as metal clips or pregnancy. It pro-

vides superior resolution of deeper structures and white matter changes. In evaluation of traumatic brain injury, the cortical contusion can be visualized by MRI after a close head injury. CT is relatively insensitive in detecting small lesions and diffuse injuries. *(Ref. 1, p. 187; Ref. 3, pp. 132–133, 433–434)*

14. **(d)** The formulation is a biopsychosocial integration of the important clinical findings that have interacted over time for a particular child or adolescent. It provides a multidimensional picture of the child that goes far beyond a recounting of the clinical history or diagnostic label, facilitating the development of a comprehensive treatment plan. *(Ref. 1, pp. 205–211; Ref. 3, pp. 539–540)*

15. **(c)** At a serum level of 1.4 mEq/L or higher, common lithium toxicity signs (such as tremor, blurred vision, ataxia, hyperreflexia, dysarthria, and diarrhea) can occur. *(Ref. 3, p. 967)*

16. **(d)** Several studies show benefits of using divalproex alone or combining with other medicines in treating bipolar disorder in youth. The recommended target serum level of divalproex is 85–110 µg/L. *(Ref. 3, pp. 967–968)*

17. **(e)** It is generally important to interview the parents first when evaluating a case of very young children. Interviewing or assessing a young child in the presence of the parents can decrease the child's anxiety, which enhances the child's performance. Observing the interactions between the child and the parents and the child's spontaneous play are important parts of the psychiatric assessment. Adolescents may be seen alone for the first interview at their request. If an adolescent is self-referred, in many states parents do not need to be notified, although it is usually advisable to insist on parental involvement in ongoing treatment. *(Ref. 1, pp. 106, 113, 117; Ref. 2, pp. 11–12; Ref. 3, pp. 527–531)*

18. **(c)** Adolescents should be reassured that specific information will be shared only with their permission, except when there is a risk of harm or abuse. Substance use may not necessarily warrant a disclosure to adolescents' parents automatically. The clinician/therapist has to make a judgment call to decide whether adolescents are engaging in significant high-risk behaviors that cause safety concerns. If so, confidentiality should be broken and the parents should be informed. Practically, skillful interviewing techniques can be used to preserve the therapist–patient alliance. When the adolescent wants to use the clinician as a "spokesperson" to inform the parents of something, the adolescent's presence is needed. *(Ref. 1, pp. 114, 217; Ref. 3, pp. 900–901)*

19. **(d)** Neurologic soft signs reflect neurodevelopmental immaturities that have persisted and often have a genetic component. They do not represent a specific neurologic or psychiatric disorder, although they do represent neurodevelopmental vulnerability and are associated with premotor frontal lobe underdevelopment or abnormal frontal lobe development. They present more frequently in some psychiatric disorders such as ADHD, schizophrenia, obsessive–compulsive disorder (OCD), and Tourette's disorder. They are more predictive of anxiety and withdrawal, but not ADHD. *(Ref. 1, p. 492; Ref. 3, pp. 573–580)*

20. **(b)** Some deficiency-related disorders, such as pellagra, can cause thought disorder, but iron deficiency is not usually a cause. In addition to the listed potential etiologies of thought disorders or hallucinations in young people, other causes to be considered include other endocrine abnormalities, seizure disorder, genetic factors, traumatic events, tumors, idiopathic factors, and psychological stress. *(Ref. 3, p. 535)*

21. **(d)** Infections such as encephalitis, meningitis, acute febrile illnesses, and brain abscesses can lead to hallucinations that are limited to the infectious period. Mononucleosis is not associated with hallucinations. *(Ref. 3, pp. 535–536)*

22. **(a)** In addition to sublimation, altruism is a more mature and higher level defense mechanism. Besides the other choices listed, projection, reaction formation, suppression, somatization, and turning passive to active are all some of the defense mechanisms that children frequently use. *(Ref. 3, pp. 199, 976–977)*

23. **(b)** Affective lability is not generally considered a positive attribute. Other positive attributes include intelligence, emotional and affective flexibility, physical fitness, psychological mindedness, good work habits and academic achievement, and appropriate ethical values. *(Ref. 3, p. 539)*

24. **(d)** The report is not usually sent to school teachers unless parents and the youth have given authorization to release the records. The parents and the child should be informed of and prepared for the conclusion of the initial phase of evaluation and included in the discussion of findings, recommendations, and the selection of a potential treatment plan. Treatment is less likely to be successful unless the parents can be engaged as allies in the treatment process. *(Ref. 1, pp. 215–218; Ref. 3, pp. 539–540)*

25. **(b)** Thyroid dysfunction can cause depression, but usually not mania. Hyperthyroidism or hypothyroidism can be seen in the other conditions listed and should be ruled out as part of the workup. Recent studies also report abnormal thyroid function may cause ADHD-like symptoms. *(Ref. 1, pp. 184–185)*

26. **(c)** The DST is reported to have a higher sensitivity in children (58%) than in adolescents (44%). Studies also show that sensitivity is higher in inpatients than in outpatients. Its specificity is better in adolescents and in inpatients. Its usage as a depression diagnostic screening tool is limited but it may still be helpful to monitor depression treatment response. *(Ref. 1, p. 450)*

27. **(d)** Wilson's disease is a recessively inherited disorder of copper metabolism but is not diagnosable by genetic techniques. Fragile X syndrome is associated with a propensity for the X chromosome to break under certain conditions, and patients have increased impulsivity and immaturity. In Turner's syndrome, 45 XO, patients have spatial processing deficits. In Klinefelter's syndrome, males have an additional X chromosome and most have verbal cognitive deficits. Prader–Willi syndrome results from absence or deletion of a function gene on chromosome 15. *(Ref. 1, pp. 186–187)*

28. **(a)** Research has reported that some neurostructural changes found in brain imaging studies are associated with certain psychiatric disorders, including ADHD, OCD, schizophrenia,

autism, and mental retardation. However, the results do not yet support the use of imaging to make these diagnoses. Imaging should be considered in children and adolescents with neurologic abnormalities suggesting increasing seizures, space-occupying lesions, certain suspected genetic syndromes, and rapid onset of psychiatric symptoms. *(Ref. 1, p. 187)*

29. **(b)** DSM-IV (DSM-IV-TR) is based on a categorical (not dimensional) classification approach. Compared to the dimensional approach, the categorical approach is more useful practically, but has less satisfactory reliability. Limitations are found in both approaches, yet certain agreements exist between them, especially for more common disorders. *(Ref. 3, pp. 501–503; Ref. 4, pp. xxxi–xxxii)*

30. **(e)** A lot of changes have been made to the text of the DSM-IV-TR for many disorders usually first diagnosed in infancy, youth, and adolescence, including information regarding specific gene mutation in Rett's disorder; an increased prevalence rate of autistic disorder; and certain etiological factors, such as fragile X syndrome, of mental retardation. No change has been made for selective mutism in the DSM-IV-TR. *(Ref. 4, pp. 829–832)*

31. **(b)** Systematically collecting and organizing information can help to eliminate bias. The other factors listed all can lead to a potentially biased diagnosis. *(Ref. 1, p. 138)*

32. **(e)** The dynamic formulation is conceptually related to psychoanalytic models and the derivative dynamic models explain behavior and emotion. The dynamic formulation provides a frame of reference to help interpret the underlying meaning of symptoms. Operant conditioning is related to behavioral (not dynamic) theories. *(Ref. 1, p. 211; Ref. 3, pp. 999–1000)*

33. **(c)** No ECG monitoring is needed when taking SSRIs, although ECG is needed if there are comorbid cardiac disease or high risk factors. A baseline ECG is indicated when using tricyclic antidepressants and for monitoring of these medications. It may be indicated for lithium and neuroleptic medications. Stimulants do not require laboratory or ECG measures for their routine use. But it may be indicated when combined with clonidine. *(Ref. 1, pp. 185, 938–943; Ref. 3, pp. 951–971)*

34. **(d)** Neurologic malignant syndrome is a potentially fatal adverse reaction to neuroleptic medication. The most common laboratory abnormalities are elevations in CPK, leukocytosis (with a shift to the left), myoglobulinuria, and occasional elevations on liver function tests. Thyroid function is not an indicator of neuroleptic malignant syndrome. Vital signs and mental status should be closely monitored. *(Ref. 1, p. 942; Ref. 2, p. 304; Ref. 3, p. 962)*

35. **(b)** An EEG is usually not indicated unless there is suspension of seizures. It is essential to evaluate for the presence of liver, kidney, hematological, and endocrine abnormalities; arrhythmias; and osteopenia, which are associated with anorexia nervosa and have potentially serious complications associated with abnormal values. Except for atypical presentations, extensive neurological evaluations or testing is not usually warranted. Computed tomography and MRI imaging studies have shown abnormal but not diagnostic findings in anorexic adolescents. *(Ref. 1, pp. 673–676; Ref. 3, pp. 692–696)*

18
CASE HISTORIES

QUESTIONS

Case 1

Andrew, a 4-year-old only child, is brought for evaluation by his White, upper-middle-class parents. His parents are seeking consultation because of Andrew's social difficulties at nursery school. Andrew does not enjoy playing with other children and has limited social interactions with them. He is described by his parents as having been a difficult baby in that he was not easily consoled and the attainment of developmental milestones was delayed. Andrew's communication is unusual in that he exhibits echolalia and monotonously repeats phrases he has heard on television. In addition, he tends to flap his hands and bang his head when he is stressed by unfamiliar circumstances and loud noises.

Questions 1–10. Based on the information given in Case 1, answer the following questions.

1. Which of the following would you *least expect* to find at the time of your initial meeting with Andrew?
   a. Andrew separates from his parents without great difficulty.
   b. He moves rapidly from toy to toy, playing with each for a few minutes.
   c. Communication is odd and idiosyncratic.
   d. His play is repetitive and stereotyped.
   e. There is limited interaction with you in the playroom.

2. Which of the following is the *most likely* DSM-IV-TR diagnosis at this point without knowing additional information?
   a. Pervasive development disorder not otherwise specified
   b. Schizophrenia
   c. Autistic disorder
   d. Reactive attachment disorder
   e. Major depressive disorder

3. Which of the following would be the *least useful* piece of additional information to help you determine the diagnosis?
   a. A complete medical history
   b. Genetic history of emotional and developmental disorders
   c. Age of onset of symptoms
   d. Course or development of the disorder
   e. History of the attainment of developmental milestones

4. At this point in your workup, which of the following is the *least likely* disorder or condition that needs to be ruled out?
   a. Asperger's syndrome
   b. Childhood disintegrative disorder
   c. Developmental language disorder
   d. Hearing impairment
   e. Mental retardation

5. Which of the following additional testing would provide the *least helpful* piece of information in treatment planning and prognosis generation?
   a. An IQ determination
   b. Determination of adaptive capabilities
   c. Standardized determination of developmental level
   d. Speech and language evaluation
   e. Magnetic resonance imaging (MRI)

6. Which of the following would you *least expect* to find with psychological and developmental testing?
   a. Below normal IQ
   b. More impairment in performance relative to abstract skills
   c. Uneven developmental attainments and levels
   d. Difficulty with sequencing and coding information
   e. Good memory skills as compared with other abilities

7. Which of the following values represents the *best* approximation to the axis V scale value of the DSM-IV-TR for Andrew?
   a. 3
   b. 15
   c. 35
   d. 55
   e. 85

8. Which of the following is the *least important* element to be included in your etiologic formulation?
   a. Genetic history
   b. IQ
   c. Speech and language attainment
   d. Family psychodynamics
   e. Adaptive abilities

9. Which of the following represents the *most important* part of Andrew's treatment plan?
   a. Individual psychotherapy
   b. Psychotropic medication
   c. Family therapy
   d. Special school placement
   e. Residential placement

10. Which of the following factors is the *least helpful* in suggesting what the prognosis for Andrew's disorder will be?
    a. His IQ
    b. History of perinatal complications
    c. Amount and quality of speech
    d. Severity of the disorder
    e. Developmental milestones

Case 2

Adam is an 8-year-old boy brought for evaluation by his single mother because of his behavioral problems at school. Adam has been having difficulties getting along with his classmates because of his aggressive behavior. His teacher has expressed concern to Adam's mother as he also has been having difficulties in academic performance. The teacher says he is "hyperactive"—shouting out answers, interrupting teachers, and being very disruptive in class. The teacher thinks Adam needs medication. Described as always on the go even as an infant, Adam reached his developmental milestones at a normal age, but has always been somewhat clumsy. Adam's father never lived with him and his mother.

Questions 11–20. Based on the information given in Case 2, answer the following questions.

11. Which of the following would you *most expect* to find during your clinical evaluation of Adam?

    a. A withdrawn child who will not leave his mother in the waiting room.
    b. A child who moves quickly from toy to toy, playing with each one briefly.
    c. A child who does not interact with you in the playroom.
    d. A child who engages in bizarre play.
    e. A child with odd and idiosyncratic communication.

12. Assuming that the answer to question 11 is b, the most likely differential diagnosis at this point should include all of the following *except:*

    a. Attention-deficit hyperactivity disorder (ADHD)
    b. Oppositional defiant disorder
    c. Obsessive–compulsive disorder
    d. Bipolar disorder
    e. Generalized anxiety disorder

13. If Adam exhibits symptoms seen in answers c, d, or e to question 11, your differential diagnosis should now include all of the following except:

    a. Pervasive developmental disorder
    b. Bipolar disorder
    c. Schizophrenic disorder
    d. Selective mutism
    e. Schizotypal personality disorder

14. Which of the following pieces of information would be *least helpful* to you in making a diagnosis?

    a. Mental health history of Adam's parents
    b. Psychological testing
    c. Academic performance history
    d. Evaluation of Adam's living environment
    e. Results from MRI or computed tomography (CT)

15. Results from which of the following assessment instruments would be the *least helpful* in establishing a DSM-IV-TR diagnosis for Adam at this point?

    a. Child Behavior Checklist (CBCL)
    b. Connor's Parent–Teacher Rating Scale
    c. ADHD Rating Scale-IV
    d. School Situation Questionnaires, Revised (SSQ-R)
    e. Minnesota Multiphasic Personality Inventory (MMPI)

16. Which of the following is the *least useful* piece of information in developing the formulation?

    a. Family history of psychiatric disorder
    b. Role of the father's absence
    c. Presence of neurologic soft signs
    d. Socioeconomic and cultural background
    e. Adaptive and coping abilities

17. Assuming that your final diagnosis is ADHD, which of the following medications would you be *least likely* to consider in the pharmacologic portion of the treatment plan?

    a. Clonidine
    b. Atomoxetine
    c. Methylphenidate
    d. Risperidone
    e. Bupropion

18. Assuming that your final diagnosis is an early thought disorder, which of the following treatment modalities is *least* indicated at this point?

    a. Environmental stabilization
    b. Psychotropic medication
    c. Family therapy
    d. Stress management
    e. Psychiatric hospitalization

19. Assuming that Adam has ADHD and you decide to use stimulant medication as part of your treatment plan, the *least likely* potential side effects of stimulant medications you might describe to Adam's mother are:

    a. Exacerbation of tics
    b. Insomnia
    c. Weight gain and growth acceleration
    d. Irritability
    e. Headache and stomachache

20. If Adam has ADHD, what is the *most likely* outcome of his disorder?

    a. Fairly normal functioning as an adult
    b. Continued problems with concentration and social, emotional, and impulse-control problems
    c. Decreased likelihood of developing major depressive disorder (MDD)
    d. Stable job status
    e. More years of school education

Case 3

Susan is a 14-year-old girl who was brought to the emergency room by her mother after Susan told her mother that she had taken an "overdose" of 10 aspirin tablets. Susan says that she took the overdose because she was angry at her older sister, who would not drive her to see a friend. At the time of evaluation in the emergency room, Susan said she regretted taking the overdose, denied feeling depressed, and said that she wanted to go home.

Questions 21–30. Based on the information given in Case 3, answer the following questions.

21. Which of the following pieces of additional information would be the *least important* for you to know in order to determine a plan for disposition?

    a. Previous suicide attempts
    b. Recent humiliating experience
    c. IQ
    d. That a friend or family member has committed suicide
    e. Presence of a psychiatric disorder

22. Which of the following is the *least likely* diagnosis that you would expect to find in your examination of Susan based on the information that you have so far?

    a. Major depressive disorder
    b. Substance abuse
    c. Borderline personality disorder
    d. Avoidant personality disorder
    e. Conduct disorder

23. All of the following findings from the psychiatric examination would indicate a greater suicide risk *except:*

    a. Absence of depressive symptoms
    b. Hopelessness
    c. Regret at being rescued
    d. Psychosis
    e. Refusal to accept help

24. All of the following findings would significantly increase the likelihood that Susan has a substance abuse problem *except:*

    a. A family history of alcoholism
    b. A history of sensation-seeking behavior
    c. Family and cultural sanctions against substance abuse
    d. A peer group that uses substances
    e. A history of psychiatric disorder

25. Disorders of impulse control, such as suicide attempts, substance abuse, and eating disorders, are *most* likely to show abnormalities in which of the following neurotransmitters?

    a. Opioids
    b. Norepinephrine
    c. Dopamine
    d. Acetylcholine
    e. Serotonin

26. In determining whether to hospitalize Susan, which of the following is the *least important* factor suggesting that outpatient treatment could be attempted?

    a. Susan's family's acceptance of the problem.
    b. Susan's absence of other comorbid psychiatric diagnoses.
    c. Susan's wish to return home.
    d. Susan's ability to promise abstention from suicide until she meets with a therapist.
    e. Susan's ability to develop a reasonable plan of action should she feel suicidal again.

27. Assuming you feel that Susan may have a substance abuse problem, which of the following would you find the *least helpful* measure of her cooperation if she were to be seen on an outpatient basis?

    a. Her cooperation with random urine screens.
    b. Her family's involvement in therapy with her.
    c. Her regular attendance at therapy and a support group.
    d. Her willingness to read educational material regarding substance abuse.
    e. Her attendance at a self-help group for substance abuse.

28. Assuming you determine that Susan has a major depressive disorder and you elect to treat her with a selective serotonin reuptake inhibitor (SSRI), which of the following tests is *most* likely to be indicated?

    a. Liver function tests
    b. Electrocardiogram (ECG)
    c. Thyroid function tests
    d. Creatinine clearance or blood urea nitrogen (BUN)
    e. Complete blood count (CBC)

29. During your psychotherapy with Susan, she develops positive and negative feelings toward you that indicate that she has developed a strong transference to you. Based on this, which of the following is the *best* course of action?

    a. Discuss with Susan transferring her to another therapist for whom she has less strong feelings.
    b. Decrease individual sessions and increase family therapy.
    c. Encourage Susan to tell you about her feelings.
    d. Explain the concepts of transference and countertransference to Susan.
    e. Discourage Susan from developing these unreasonable feelings.

30. The *most hopeful* prognostic sign in the information presented about Susan is that:

    a. She wants to go home.
    b. She took only 10 aspirin tablets.
    c. She says that she is not depressed.
    d. She told her mother of her attempt and her mother took her to the emergency room.
    e. She expressed regret at taking the overdose.

Case 4

Beth is a 14-year-old girl who was hospitalized on the pediatric ward after her diabetes got out of control and she developed keto-acidosis. The request from pediatrics for psychiatric consultation states: "Patient is a management problem. Please advise."

Questions 31–40. Based on the information given in Case 4, answer the following questions.

31. Based on this limited information, your *first* step should be to:
   a. Send the consult request form back with a note to the effect that there is insufficient information.
   b. Read the patient's chart.
   c. Talk to the nurses on the floor where the patient is hospitalized.
   d. Call the referring pediatrician and ask for more information about the request.
   e. See the patient.

32. You learn that Beth was first diagnosed as having juvenile-onset diabetes mellitus in childhood, which was under good control until she entered adolescence, when she became non-compliant with diet, urine checks, and dosage adjustments. She has been in the hospital five times in the past year with severe ketoacidosis. Based on this, the *most likely* explanation for her behavior is:
   a. Her diabetes has become more difficult to control as a result of hormonal variations.
   b. The frequent episodes of ketoacidosis represent disguised suicide attempts.
   c. Her difficulty with controlling her diabetes represents a struggle with tasks of adolescent development.
   d. Her physician is mismanaging her.
   e. Beth has a psychiatric disorder.

33. You learn that Beth has markedly decreased potassium and increased serum amylase on a regular basis. When you mention this to the patient's attending, she says that she suspects that the patient may be bingeing and vomiting. The patient is 5 feet, 5 inches tall, and she weighs 100 pounds, with normal menstrual periods. The *most likely* diagnosis in the following differential is:
   a. Bulimia nervosa
   b. Anorexia nervosa
   c. Prader–Willi syndrome
   d. Psychogenic vomiting
   e. Generalized anxiety disorder

34. Additional evaluation leads you to believe that the patient has bulimia nervosa and is self-inducing vomiting. When you share this with the attending pediatrician, the doctor becomes very angry at the patient for "causing" her life-threatening illness. Which of the following interactions with the pediatrician is likely to be the *least helpful* to Beth in the long run?
   a. Offering to take over the management of the case.
   b. Offering to be part of Beth's treatment team on pediatrics.
   c. Explaining the developmental nature of Beth's disorder.
   d. Offering clear suggestions for working effectively with Beth.
   e. Determining the source of the pediatrician's anger.

35. The nursing staff members on the floor where Beth is hospitalized are "split" as to how they regard Beth. Some like her very much and defend her, and the others are very angry with her and critical of her. Which of the following suggestions is likely to be the *least helpful* to Beth and the nursing staff?
   a. Designating a team of nurses to work with Beth.
   b. Instituting a postmeal watch with a nurse and Beth.
   c. Meeting daily with the team of nurses working with Beth.
   d. Pointing out to the nurses that their anger at or defense of Beth has to do with their own control issues.
   e. Providing the nursing staff with reading material about eating disorders.

36. You meet with Beth's parents. Her father is a successful politician in the community, and is often away from the home. Her mother is an attorney who stopped practicing several years earlier so that she could be at home with Beth. You sense that there is a great deal of marital conflict, and that it is causing Beth distress. Which of the following is likely to be the *least helpful* suggestion to the parents?
   a. Asking to meet with the family again while Beth is in the hospital.
   b. Asking for permission to talk with the family doctor to gather further information.
   c. Suggesting that the mother go to work and that the father spend more time at home.
   d. Suggesting that the family may benefit from family therapy.
   e. Suggesting to the family that emotional stress can exacerbate physical disorders.

37. In your fourth meeting with Beth, she confides in you that her father has been sexually molesting her for several months. The molestation consists of genital fondling in her bed late at night and has not involved penetration. Which of the following possible actions is the *most appropriate?*
   a. Notify the attending pediatrician and report to authorities immediately.
   b. Notify the patient's father that the suspected child abuse will be reported to authorities.
   c. Gather further information before notifying the authorities.
   d. Allow Beth to return home with her father before further evaluation or investigation.
   e. Continue the evaluation without notifying the authorities since penetration did not occur.

38. Based on this new information, Beth is at risk of having or developing all of the following disorders. Which is the *least likely?*
   a. Posttraumatic stress disorder (PTSD)

b. Somatization disorder

c. Substance abuse disorder

d. Major depressive disorder

e. Conduct disorder

39. Which of the following considerations is the *least important* in considering whether or when to arrange for Beth to be transferred to a psychiatric unit?

a. Beth's medical condition is stable enough to be managed on the psychiatric unit.

b. The psychiatric unit agrees to manage Beth's medical condition.

c. Beth agrees to the transfer to the psychiatric unit.

d. The parents agree to the transfer to the psychiatric unit.

e. The attending pediatrician agrees to the transfer to the psychiatric unit.

40. Based on the combination of Beth's disorders, which of the following is the *most likely* prognosis?

a. Beth will not have significant psychiatric difficulties in the future.

b. Beth will be overly concerned with food and weight and her sexuality, but will live a fairly "normal" life.

c. Beth will have episodic psychiatric disability during times of stress and is at increased risk of depressive disorders.

d. Beth will have chronic psychiatric disability and is at increased risk of suicide.

e. It is too early to say for certain whether Beth will do well or do poorly.

ANSWERS AND EXPLANATIONS

Case 1

1. (b) Andrew's presentation so far most resembles one of the pervasive developmental disorders. Based on this, you would expect to find limitations in reciprocal social interactions, verbal and nonverbal communication, and imaginative activities; cognitive deficits; and repetitive, ritualistic activities. Moving rapidly from toy to toy and playing briefly with each would be unusual for a child with pervasive developmental disorder, and would be more characteristic of a child with ADHD or psychosocial deprivation or disorganization. *(Ref. 1, pp. 261–269; Ref. 3, pp. 587–591)*

2. (a) While Andrew's presentation so far has features of autistic disorder, he does not seem to have enough symptoms or severe enough symptoms to meet the full criteria for autistic disorder. In this case, pervasive developmental disorder not otherwise specified (PDDNOS) is the most appropriate diagnosis. Childhood schizophrenia is ruled out by the absence of reported hallucinations or delusions and the age and nature of onset. Reactive attachment disorder is ruled out by the nature of the reported interaction with primary caretakers and the communication and social interactive style. *(Ref. 1, pp. 261–271, 338–341; Ref. 3, pp. 588–589; Ref. 4, pp. 69–75, 84)*

3. (b) Autistic disorders have a genetic and biologic basis, but a genetic history of emotional or developmental disorders does not help in determining the diagnosis from the possibilities. Certain medical conditions are associated with pervasive developmental disorders and with disorders that can be confused with autistic disorders. A complete medical history and the age of onset and course of the disorder are the most useful pieces of history to determine the diagnosis. *(Ref. 1, pp. 274–288; Ref. 3, pp. 591–592)*

4. (d) Hearing impairment is important to be ruled out in the evaluation of younger children who present with delayed development of language, but it is unlikely in Andrew's case based on his age and presentation. All of the other disorders listed cannot be ruled out based on the information given so far. *(Ref. 1, pp. 269–273; Ref. 3, pp. 588–589, 593; Ref. 4, pp. 74)*

5. (e) Research studies have shown neurostructural changes associated with autistic disorder, but the significance of these for outcome or treatment is not yet known. The IQ and areas of strength and weakness developmentally and in speech and language would all be useful in determining the treatment plan and the prognosis. *(Ref. 1, pp. 279–293; Ref. 3, pp. 590–594; Ref. 4, p. 73)*

6. (b) Children with pervasive developmental disorder, especially autism, have greater difficulty with verbal and abstract abilities and do relatively better on performance portions, such as immediate memory and visual–spatial skills. *(Ref. 1, pp. 266–267; Ref. 3, pp. 590–591)*

7. (d) Axis V is the Global Assessment of Functioning Scale (GAF scale) of the DSM-IV-TR and can range from 0 to 100. While there is some variability in the way in which clinicians rate individuals on this scale, one should be able to get into an expected range. Axis IV is psychosocial and environmental problems and is grouped by problem categories. Based on the information given, Andrew falls into a score of around 50 to 60, which represents moderate to serious symptoms and impairment in social and school settings. *(Ref. 4, pp. 32–34)*

8. (d) Family coping abilities are important to consider in the formulation, but usually have little to do with the etiology of pervasive developmental disorder. Family psychodynamics should not be dismissed and are important in treatment planning, but are relatively less important in determining the etiology than the other pieces of information listed. *(Ref. 1, pp. 274–288; Ref. 3, pp. 591–592)*

9. (d) Educational interventions to enhance social, cognitive, and communicative skills represent the most helpful intervention for pervasive developmental disorder. Residential placement is usually not necessary with younger children. Individual and family therapy can be useful in reducing secondary psychological complications. No psychotropic medications have been found to be clearly helpful for the core symptoms of this disorder, but they may be helpful for concurrent disorders and symptoms associated with this disorder. *(Ref. 1, pp. 288–295; Ref. 3, pp. 593–594)*

10. (b) Predictors of good outcome include higher IQ, better language skills, later onset, and less severe symptoms. Perinatal complications may help with the etiology, but are not by themselves helpful in determining the prognosis. *(Ref. 1, pp. 295–296; Ref. 3, p. 594)*

Case 2

11. (b) Based on the information provided so far, Adam seems most likely to have a behavioral disturbance such as ADHD or possibly oppositional defiant disorder or conduct disorder. You would most likely expect Adam to move quickly from toy to toy rather than to be withdrawn, emotionally aloof, or bizarre. *(Ref. 1, pp. 488–491; Ref. 3, pp. 647–650; Ref. 4, pp. 85–88)*

12. (c) The symptoms presented are most consistent with an externalizing disorder such as ADHD, oppositional defiant disorder, or conduct disorder. Generalized anxiety disorder and mood disorders should also be considered. Obsessive–compulsive disorder is very unlikely based on the information given. *(Ref. 1, pp. 491–492; Ref. 3, pp. 651–655; Ref. 4, p. 91)*

13. (d) Difficulties with attention and impulse control are often early signs of schizophrenic disorder and bipolar disorder, and may also be seen in pervasive developmental disorder and schizotypal personality disorder. The information given so far makes selective mutism the most unlikely diagnosis. *(Ref. 1, pp. 491–492; Ref. 3, pp. 361, 651–655; Ref. 4, p. 91)*

14. **(e)** Based on the history, which indicates a chronic, nonprogressive disorder, it is unlikely that Adam has a space-occupying or neurodegenerative lesion that would make brain imaging useful. Brain imaging is still more valuable in research settings than in making psychiatric diagnoses in clinical settings. *(Ref. 1, pp. 493–495; Ref. 3, pp. 650–651)*

15. **(e)** The MMPI does not lead to a DSM-IV diagnosis, nor does it evaluate specifically for behavior disorders in childhood. The CBCL, Connor's, ADHD Rating Scale-IV, and the School Situations Questionnaires, Revised, could all provide useful information to help determine the severity of externalizing behavior, such as ADHD and oppositional defiant disorder. *(Ref. 1, pp. 149–154; Ref. 3, pp. 559, 565–566, 650–656)*

16. **(c)** Neurologic soft signs are indicative of neurodevelopmental immaturity and/or dysfunction and are associated with a wide variety of disorders, including ADHD and schizophrenic disorders. Their presence may add support to the role of genetic and biologic vulnerability, but they are not as useful as the other pieces of information listed. *(Ref. 1, pp. 492–494; Ref. 3, pp. 577–578, 650–657)*

17. **(d)** Neuroleptic medications such as risperidone are not indicated in the treatment of ADHD except in severely ill children who are not responding to other choices. Approximately 75% of children will respond to the first stimulant medication; 90% who did not respond to the first stimulant medication will respond to an alternative. Atomoxetine and antidepressants should be considered if there are affective or anxious symptoms or if side effects are a problem with stimulant medication. Clonidine should also be considered when side effects of stimulants are a problem. Clonidine improves frustration tolerance and compliance, but does not increase attention or decrease distractibility. *(Ref. 1, pp. 495–498; Ref. 3, pp. 659–661)*

18. **(e)** None of the symptoms described so far indicate a need for psychiatric hospitalization. It has been suggested, but not experimentally demonstrated, that low doses of neuroleptic may improve the long-term prognosis for children at high risk for developing a thought disorder. All of the other modalities are clearly indicated to help the child and the family manage stress, and thus "protect" against the risk of inducing a psychotic decompensation. *(Ref. 1, pp. 399–402; Ref. 3, pp. 751–753)*

19. **(c)** Stimulant medications in the treatment of children with ADHD can result in some potential side effects, such as appetite and growth suppression, weight loss, exacerbation of tics, emotional lability and irritability, headache, stomachache, insomnia, fatigue, skin picking, and, rarely, psychosis. *(Ref. 1, pp. 496–497, 932–935; Ref. 2, pp. 272–276; Ref. 3, pp. 660–661)*

20. **(b)** According to the long-term outcome studies that exist, as children with ADHD become adults they continue to show significant impairment in a number of aspects of their lives. A significant percentage of adults with a previous diagnosis of ADHD continue to experience disabling ADHD symptoms.

In addition, they have fewer years of school education, a less stable job history, and a greater chance of being diagnosed with MDD. *(Ref. 1, p. 500; Ref. 3, pp. 664–665)*

Case 3

21. **(c)** The IQ is not a predictor of youth suicidal behavior. Predictors of suicidal risk are previous suicide attempts; recent stresses, including a humiliating experience; the effects of modeling or contagion; psychiatric disorders; social functioning; and biological factors. *(Ref. 1, pp. 897–898; Ref. 3, pp. 798–801)*

22. **(d)** The most common psychiatric diagnoses found in adolescents who attempt suicide include depressive disorders, conduct disorder, substance abuse, and other personality disorders associated with poor impulse control, such as borderline personality disorder. Avoidant personality disorder has not been associated with suicide. Bisexual or homosexual adolescents also have a higher risk for attempting suicide. *(Ref. 1, pp. 897–898; Ref. 2, p. 214; Ref. 3, pp. 798–799)*

23. **(a)** Because presence of a depressive disorder increases a risk of suicide, it is important to inquire about depressive symptoms during the suicide evaluation. It is not unusual for adolescents to deny depressive feelings, although symptoms of depression usually can be elicited by direct questioning about neurovegetative symptoms, such as sleep and appetite disturbance, difficulties in concentrating, loss of interests, and hopelessness. *(Ref. 1, pp. 897–898; Ref. 2, p. 214; Ref. 3, pp. 798–799)*

24. **(c)** Genetic, parental, individual, and sociocultural factors all play a role in the etiology of substance abuse. Studies indicate that sociocultural sanctions against substance abuse decrease the likelihood of abuse. *(Ref. 1, p. 800; Ref. 3, pp. 896–898)*

25. **(e)** Serotonin and norepinephrine are dysfunctional in eating disorders and depression. Serotonin also has been shown to play a role in disruptive behaviors with poor impulse control. *(Ref. 3, pp. 53–54, 389, 800)*

26. **(c)** Susan's desire to go home is of little value in determining her future suicidal risk (e.g., she could feel humiliated if she does not return home, increasing risk, or she could want to go home to make a more serious attempt). Her ability to promise abstention from suicidal behavior until seen by a professional may not guarantee abstention, but her reaction to making the promise often reveals underlying motivations. *(Ref. 1, p. 899; Ref. 3, p. 803)*

27. **(d)** There is little indication that educational approaches by themselves are helpful in treating substance abuse. The commitment of Susan and her family to treatment is probably the best positive predictor. *(Ref. 1, pp. 800–805; Ref. 3, pp. 901–907)*

28. **(c)** The most important rule-out and baseline in treating MDD with an SSRI is a thyroid function test because thyroid dysfunction is associated with mood disorders, anxiety disorders, and, rarely, psychosis. It is not routinely indicated and should be considered only if symptoms or physical exam suggests it is indicated. *(Ref. 1, pp. 183–185; Ref. 3, pp. 106–107)*

29. (c) At times it may be appropriate to explain the concepts of transference and countertransference to an adolescent patient, but it should be done cautiously to avoid the risk of intellectualizing the feelings or scaring the patient away. The best course is to encourage Susan's expression of feelings and to examine transference and countertransference issues yourself. The feeling of rejection involved in transferring Susan to another therapist or decreasing her sessions in favor of family therapy could be detrimental to Susan. *(Ref. 1, p. 859; Ref. 3, pp. 975, 978, 987)*

30. (d) The fact that Susan told her mother of her attempt and that her mother took her to the emergency room indicates that the mother and Susan have enough of a potential relationship to be involved in therapy together. In the determination of the potential lethality of a suicide attempt, it is important to determine the belief that the method could result in death rather than its actual lethality. As discussed earlier, depressed adolescents initially may deny feelings of depression. Expressions of regret may be a good prognostic sign, but may also represent a way to get out of the emergency room. *(Ref. 1, pp. 897–899; Ref. 3, pp. 799–803)*

Case 4

31. (d) The most important first step in providing a consultation is to determine what question is being asked, either directly or indirectly, by those requesting the consultation. All of the other steps listed are important to take, but not until you have determined why the consult is being requested. *(Ref. 3, p. 1114)*

32. (c) While all of the responses are possibilities to be considered, the most likely explanation for Beth's increased difficulties in controlling her diabetes is that she is struggling with issues of dependence and independence through defensive functions, such as denial, reaction formation, and counterphobia. *(Ref. 3, p. 1235)*

33. (a) In Prader–Willi syndrome, a genetic disorder, the patient may binge and is very short and grossly overweight. Anorexia nervosa is unlikely because of the patient's weight and normal menstrual periods. Bulimia nervosa seems the most likely possibility, but the possibility that the patient vomits as a result of anxiety or other psychogenic causes must be explored. *(Ref. 1, pp. 671–675, 692–700; Ref. 3, pp. 692–696)*

34. (a) Beth's medical disorder will need continued management. Interrupting her primary relationship with her pediatrician at this point is likely to be harmful for Beth in the long run. Explaining the developmental nature of her disorder must be done in a manner that does not seem condescending to the pediatrician, or this approach could also be damaging. *(Ref. 3, pp. 1116–1119)*

35. (d) Offering an interpretation before sufficient rapport is established is likely to alienate the nurses, and could increase their anger at you and Beth. *(Ref. 3, pp. 1117–1119)*

36. (c) There are potential problems with answers **b** and **d**, but answer **c** has the clearest possibility of alienating the family with unsolicited advice, especially before establishing a therapeutic relationship. The family may feel threatened by the request to seek additional information from the family doctor, but this approach may serve as a bridge to help them get into therapy. The direct suggestion of the need for family therapy may need to come after another meeting with the family. *(Ref. 1, pp. 125–133; Ref. 3, pp. 1374–1379)*

37. (a) Psychiatrists are mandatory reporters by all states. Notifying the attending pediatrician and reporting the suspected child abuse to authorities immediately is the most appropriate thing to do first. The patient will be maintained safely in the hospital while further evaluations and investigation are undertaken. It will be up to authorities to determine whether she is safe to go back to her parents after she is discharged from the hospital. *(Ref. 1, pp. 910, 915; Ref. 2, p. 224; Ref. 3, pp. 1214–1215)*

38. (e) As a result of sexual abuse, girls are likely to develop PTSD, somatization disorder, substance abuse disorder, or major depressive disorder. Conduct disorder is also a possibility, but is less likely. Sexually abused boys are likely to develop PTSD, substance abuse disorder and/or conduct disorder, and are less likely than girls to develop major depression. *(Ref. 1, pp. 861–863; Ref. 3, pp. 1218–1219)*

39. (c) While it is desirable that Beth be in favor of the transfer, her agreement is probably the least important of the possibilities listed. The psychiatric unit must agree to manage her diabetes with the consultation of pediatrics. The attending pediatrician must agree that Beth is medically ready to be transferred, and agree to have her followed on the psychiatric unit. If the parents do not cooperate with the transfer to psychiatry, therapy and discharge of Beth become very difficult. *(Ref. 3, pp. 1091–1094, 1113–1115)*

40. (e) In the long run, however, answers **c** and **d** should prove to be the most likely. Based on the limited amount of information available regarding Beth's coping abilities and early life experiences, it is probably too early to say for certain what her prognosis will be. However, based on the probabilities of the outcomes from bulimia nervosa and sexual abuse, Beth's prognosis is fair at best, and may be poor. *(Ref. 1, pp. 702, 861–863; Ref. 3, pp. 698, 1218–1221)*